Praise for *Blessing the Hands That Feed Us*

"Vicki Robin's *Blessing the Hands that Feed Us* is part how-to manual for eating 'hyperlocal' in an era where we can eat whatever we want at any time of day and part homage to the farmers around the globe who grow our food. I'm inspired not only by Robin's commitment to her own diet, but also her ability to tell the story meal by meal and farmer by farmer about why we should all be looking more closely at our own diets."
  —Danielle Nierenberg, cofounder of Food Tank: The Food Think Tank

"Whether you're a vegan, vegetarian, or eat some meat, this book can show you how and why to include 'local' on your list of important food values. Discovering the food of your bioregion, meeting your local farmers, sharing meals with friends, building community through food—all of this is part of personal and planetary health."
            —John Robbins, author *Diet for a New America* and cofounder
            of The Food Revolution Network

"Vicki Robin is modeling a self-reliant lifestyle that can end the violence our industrial food system exacts against our health, our communities, our ecosystems. It serves as a compelling manifesto of localization. An engaging, delightfully enjoyable read."
  —Michael H. Shuman, author of *Local Dollars, Local Sense: How to Move Your Money from Wall Street to Main Street and Achieve Real Prosperity*

"Vicki Robin knows that honest, engaging food writing isn't really about food. It's about friends, family, community, spirit, and soil. It's about joy. This book gracefully contains all six in equal measure."
              —Ben Hewitt, author of *The Town That Food Saved: How
              One Community Found Vitality in Local Food*

"Want to find your way from the highway of overeating to the garden of relational eating? Of course you do. For decades, Vicki Robin has been out front, showing us a new path that is not dependent upon mindless consumption. She has kept right on going, all the way to her local food system. And what a hopeful, healthy destination she has found, for her and for everyone who wants to truly and beautifully take our country forward."
                    —Woody Tasch, chairman, Slow Money

"A deeply personal and fun read that manages to both playfully and honestly recount one woman's journey into reconnection—with food, with community, and with the land itself that feeds us."
            —Nina Simons, cofounder and president, Bioneers/Collective
            Heritage Institute

"What a beautiful, honest, relatable book Vicki Robin has written. After reading it, I can't help but rethink how I eat, where I shop, and ways to do it all differently. *Blessing the Hands That Feed Us* really is a blessing to us all."
            —Geneen Roth, author of *Women, Food and God* and *Lost and Found*

"Vicki Robin has made an illuminating experiment that could help lead us all closer to a sustainable world. I especially love the way she weaves global issues into very personal, intimate stories of her own experience."
            —Starhawk, author of *The Spiral Dance*

"[*Blessing the Hands That Feed Us* is] about discovering, with gusto, the other end of the industrial food scale and how eating closer to home can affect global issues of hunger, justice, and nutrition. This enjoyable and enlightening book includes practical tips for adopting a locally sourced diet, recipes, and stories about individuals who epitomize a sustainable lifestyle."
            —*Taste for Life*

PENGUIN BOOKS

BLESSING THE HANDS THAT FEED US

Vicki Robin is a renowned innovator, writer, and speaker. In addition to coauthoring the bestselling *Your Money or Your Life*, Robin has been at the forefront of the sustainable living movement. She has received awards from Co-Op America and Sustainable Northwest and was a speaker on relational eating at TEDxSeattle. She lives on Whidbey Island in Washington.

Frances Moore Lappé is the author or coauthor of eighteen books, including the national bestseller *Diet for a Small Planet* and *EcoMind*.

Anna Lappé is the author or coauthor of three books, most recently the national bestseller *Diet for a Hot Planet: The Climate Crisis at the End of Your Fork and What You Can Do About It*.

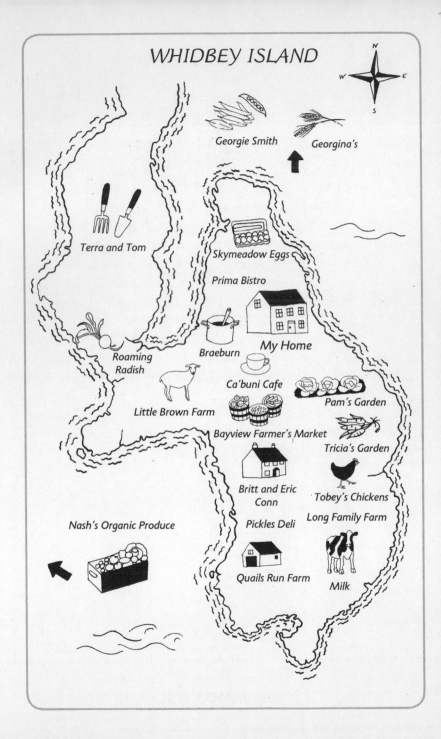

WHIDBEY ISLAND

Georgie Smith

Georgina's

Terra and Tom

Skymeadow Eggs

Prima Bistro

My Home

Braeburn

Roaming Radish

Ca'buni Cafe

Pam's Garden

Little Brown Farm

Bayview Farmer's Market

Tricia's Garden

Britt and Eric Conn

Tobey's Chickens

Long Family Farm

Nash's Organic Produce

Pickles Deli

Quails Run Farm

Milk

Blessing the Hands That Feed Us

Lessons from a 10-Mile Diet

VICKI ROBIN

PENGUIN BOOKS

PENGUIN BOOKS

Published by the Penguin Group
Penguin Group (USA) LLC
375 Hudson Street
New York, New York 10014

USA | Canada | UK | Ireland | Australia | New Zealand | India | South Africa | China
penguin.com
A Penguin Random House Company

First published in the United States of America by Viking Penguin,
a member of Penguin Group (USA) LLC, 2014
Published in Penguin Books 2014

THE LIBRARY OF CONGRESS HAS CATALOGED THE HARDCOVER EDITION AS FOLLOWS:

Robin, Vicki.
Blessing the hands that feed us : what eating closer to home can teach us about food, community, and our
place on earth / Vicki Robin.
p.   cm.
Preface by Frances Moore Lappé and Anna Lappé.
Includes bibliographical references and index.
ISBN 978-0-670-02572-5 (hc.)
ISBN 978-0-14-312614-0 (pbk.)
1. Local foods—Washington (State)—Whidbey Island. 2. Community-supported agriculture—Washington
(State)—Whidbey Island. 3. Self-reliant living—Washington (State)—Whidbey Island. 4. Whidbey Island
(Wash.)—Social conditions. I. Lappé, Frances Moore. II. Lappé, Anna, 1973– III. Title.
HD9007.W2R63 2014
363.809797′75—dc23
2013018397

Printed in the United States of America
10   9   8   7   6   5   4   3   2   1

Frontispiece map illustration by Rosie Scott

Set in Agfa Wile with Agilita and Lake Informal display
Designed by Carla Bolte

I dedicate this book to all the children born just about now. May you have green growing things outside your door. May you flourish in a garden world. May you have plenty to eat. May our generations have done something simple and good for you through encouraging sustainable agriculture and thriving local communities.

Preface

It is from numberless diverse acts of courage and belief that human history is shaped. Each time a man stands up for an ideal, or acts to improve the lot of others, or strikes out against injustice, he sends forth a tiny ripple of hope.

—Robert F. Kennedy

Vicki Robin takes the world personally and, because of that, passionately engages in questioning assumptions and searching for new ways of seeing the world that suggest new ways of being. And in this way, we see ourselves in her. Being this way in the world isn't always comfortable. It means finding yourself at cross purposes with the powers that be or at odds with received wisdom, but Vicki's writing, and this beautiful new book, allows us to experience the joy of a lifelong practice of asking questions.

When I wrote *Diet for a Small Planet* over forty years ago, I was a kid with a question: *Why are people still going hungry?* I believed that if I could figure that out, I'd have direction. At the time, the Vietnam War raged, the National Guard shot students for protesting, and discrimination was still rampant despite new civil rights laws. I was lost. I desperately wanted to help make things better, but I needed a theory of *why*, some notion of how we got into this mess, some idea of the root causes.

Then my twentysomething intuition kicked in. I suspected that since food is among our most basic human needs, grasping the whys and hows of hunger might unlock the whole mystery of economics and politics. So I set out on a quest, not to write a book, but to find the truth and share it with friends.

Soon I discovered that more than enough food was then being produced for each of us. And today it's even truer, with 2,800 calories produced for every person every year—at least a fifth more food per capita than in the late 60s. We are living in a *story* of scarcity, but not a *reality* of scarcity! I believed that once we released ourselves from the false fear of scarcity, we could get down to the real business: remaking the social and economic rules that concentrate wealth and power, making hunger inevitable no matter how much we grow.

Meanwhile, Vicki Robin was questioning another assumption: *Does stuff make us happy?* With her partner, Joe Dominguez, she scrutinized the link between money and fulfillment in the petri dish of her own life and noticed how unhooking money from happiness revealed the entrapment of "too-muchness" and the empowerment of "enoughness." They understood money as one's "life energy" and saw how investing life energy in relationships, competencies, community, and spirituality produced real wealth. Eventually they taught their radical approach in *Your Money or Your Life*.

Needless to say, the ensuing four decades haven't seen the remaking of the human story we'd imagined. Today the number of hungry people worldwide is almost exactly where it was in the 1960s. And our fear-driven culture prods us to stay within the tribe through "common purchases" rather than bonding through common purposes.

The interlocking global challenges appear far more complex and contradictory than our younger minds anticipated. And it's easy to feel so overwhelmed with fear and loss that one wonders how new ideas and new connections can possibly break through. So as the decades have passed, I've come to ask myself just one question, How do I keep the channel within me open—the channel of life's incessant insistence on *more life*?

Vicki helps me stay focused on that question. She and I actually met face-to-face nearly fifteen years ago at that moment when we were both recognizing the immensity of the challenges and both seeking a deeper understanding of what holds the old systems in place—even when we can see what's wrong and solutions are everywhere.

Twelve years ago, I joined forces with my daughter, Anna, to pick up the questions raised three decades earlier in *Diet for a Small Planet*— and we join our voices here to share the rest of our story and how it relates to Vicki's new book.

We wanted to know: Where in the world could we find communities showing new models for knitting together community, economics, and food systems so all were fed and nature's resources were treasured, not plundered. To answer this question, we traveled together to five continents and witnessed how behind the headlines and statistics about hunger and environmental devastation a globally grounded transformation is welling up. It is arising on every continent, from the neighborhood, village, town, city, and even some parliaments and global forums.

Our journey changed us forever.

Aldous Huxley wrote that "all that we are and will and do depends, in the last analysis, on what we believe the Nature of Things to be." And we came to see that our collective understanding of the Nature of Things is shifting. We humans are shedding the failed and false view that we are isolated "atoms," and with it the depressing idea that we're all essentially self-interested and selfish. We saw the evidence in community after community of the profoundly social nature of human beings.

On our journey, we met so many people starting from this experience-based—and also science-based—understanding of humanity: that our species' deepest needs are for connection, meaning, and efficacy (having a say and knowing we can make a difference). And that it is embedded in who we are to perceive our self-interest in the well-being of our communities.

Tapping these deep needs, and capacities, is just what's needed now to turn our planet toward life.

In this important new work, Vicki expresses this uplifting understanding of what it means to be human and our sense that food is a powerful avenue for engagement in a healthier and happier future.

Vicki's new work captures and furthers a movement grounded in what we think of as eyes-wide-open hope. She captures here one of our "aha" moments from our world journey. Whether expressed in Hindu farmers in India saving and saving seeds, Muslim farmers in Niger turning back the desert, or Christian farmers in the United States practicing biblically inspired Creation Care, the revolutionary power of the food is its capacity to upend a life-destroying belief system that's brought us power-concentrating corporatism.

Corporatism, after all, depends on our belief in the fairy tale that the market works on its own without us. The global, diverse, citizen-driven food movement breaks that spell—shifting our sense of self: from passive, disconnected consumers in a magical market to active, richly connected coproducers in societies we are ourselves creating— as share owners in a CSA farm or purchasers of fair trade products or actors in public life shaping the next farm bill.

Food's power is connection itself. Corporatism distances us from one another, from the earth—and even from our own bodies—while the food movement celebrates our reconnection. Years ago in Madison, Wisconsin, CSA farmer Barb Perkins said that her most rewarding moments are "like in town yesterday," she said, "I saw this little kid, wide-eyed, grab his mom's arm and point at me. 'Mommy,' he said, 'look. There's our farmer!'"

To us, this story captures Vicki's great term, "relational eating."

Food, making us aware of the power of our choices, encourages us to "think like an ecosystem," enabling us to see a place for ourselves connected to all others. For in ecological systems, "there are no parts, only participants," German physicist Hans Peter Duerr reminds us.

Blessing the Hands That Feed Us suggests that it is possible for us all to be nourished by a regional diet by feeling the relationships embodied in our food. Of course, you may be familiar with the experts who pooh-pooh such ideas, dismissing as naïve the notion that organic, regional foods can feed the world. We like to remind those so-called experts that a food system increasingly controlled by a handful of corporations is doing a decidedly poor job of feeding us, and will only become less able to do so. Almost 870 million people are suffering severe and chronic undernourishment; and obesity and overweight, linked to corporate-propagated, addictive high-calorie-low-nutrition food is the fifth leading risk factor for global deaths. We know that in aligning food and farming with nature's genius, there can be more than enough for all.

As we have encountered—and as this book shares—another way of eating and being *is* working, opening the door to perhaps the most important lessons of all about hope.

For starters, it's not for wimps: Hope is not wishful thinking. Real hope lives in our whole bodies and that only happens when we put our whole bodies into it. This is what Vicki is showing us. Hope has become for us an action verb, not a state of being, but motion itself—moving one's life day by day ever more into alignment with the world we want, ever more into alignment with what we know can meet our truest, deepest needs. And that means taking risks, risking failure and frustration, and more . . . and yet not giving up. It means knowing that we are moving shoulder to shoulder with hundreds of millions of other risk takers, the planet over, in the most exhilarating and consequential walk our species has ever taken.

All of us are in very good company as we join Vicki in learning rich lessons from a simple experiment of eating closer to home.

Frances Moore Lappé and Anna Lappé

Cambridge, Massachusetts, and Berkeley, California

Frances Moore Lappé is the author of *Diet for a Small Planet* and *Eco-Mind: Changing the Way We Think to Change the World We Want*. Anna Lappé is the author of *Diet for a Hot Planet* and the director of the Food MythBusters Initiative. Together, they wrote *Hope's Edge* and cofounded the Small Planet Institute.

Contents

Preface by
Frances Moore Lappé and Anna Lappé | ix

Introduction | 1

Chapter One   Localize Me? | 11

Chapter Two   Putting My Mouth Where My Mouth Is | 28

Chapter Three   Yes! But How? | 56

Chapter Four   Week One: Grounded! | 88

Chapter Five   Week Two: Getting the Hang of It | 111

Chapter Six   Week Three: The Week of My Discontent | 148

Chapter Seven   Revelations of the Final Week | 187

Chapter Eight   Relational Eating | 223

Chapter Nine   Bringing Our Eating Closer to Home | 261

Epilogue   Continued Blessing | 311

Acknowledgments | 319

Notes | 321
Index | 325

I begin with the proposition that eating is an agricultural act. Eating ends the annual drama of the food economy that begins with planting and birth. Most eaters, however, are no longer aware that this is true. They think of food as an agricultural product, perhaps, but they do not think of themselves as participants in agriculture. They think of themselves as "consumers."

—Wendell Berry, "The Pleasures of Eating,"
December 10, 2009, *The Contrary Farmer Blog*

"Local food? In New York all food is local. You go down to the street and it's right there."

—Phyllis Wertzl (Vicki Robin's alter ego)

Introduction

In September 2010, I undertook an experiment that turned out to be one of the greatest adventures of my life. It was so small at the start, but it eventually grew—and blew me wide open.

A farmer friend wanted a guinea pig to test whether she could actually feed another human being for a full month from what she could grow on her half acre. I wanted to test, from a sustainability perspective, if we here on Whidbey Island could survive without access to that cornucopia called the grocery store. We called the experiment a 10-mile diet.

I've done other "sustainability as an extreme sport" experiments many times. I've fasted—from food for ten days, from talking for a month, from air travel for a year—anything that would bring me closer to a life of integrity. I think sustainability is meant to be put into practice, not just debated.

The 10-mile diet was simply the next in the series. I did this experiment in hyperlocal eating wholeheartedly in September 2010, on Whidbey Island in Puget Sound in the Pacific Northwest. Whidbey is a gentle place. The island connects to the mainland via a twice-hourly ferry to the south and a bridge to the north, so our culture here is rural with an urban flair. Our climate is moderate. Driving up the long midisland highway, you might think—and tourists do—that it's a bucolic and bountiful land with a few cities strung like precious pearls on a long chain. True, but there is much more to the story.

Almost all of our daily fare comes in on semitrucks on those ferries. Our grocery stores, apparently stocked to the gills, have only a three-day supply of food. If energy prices double again—as they have in the past decade—our transport-dependent pantry might get pretty bare. But what about all that rolling farmland? Some of those crops are for export off island. Some are to feed our animals. Not everyone who owns a farm, farms. What the owners do with their land is up to them, and many who can afford big spreads don't need farming income. Then there is the wild card called climate change. Will the crops that grow well on Whidbey now grow well in the future? This year we had a late blooming summer and then months without rain. At the moment that's a pity for the farmers but not for consumers. Our "local" suppliers are not from here. Grocers buy from whoever has a reliable supply—which could be Thailand or Chile or New Zealand.

Only some Charles Addams ghoulish character would contemplate these uncertainties with delight. Most of us simply don't want to contemplate these conditions at all. After all, what can we do about it? This for me is where the "extreme sport" comes in, the real life game of skillfully reshaping assumptions and choices in light of the most likely scenarios. I know that change can be rapid, unpredictable, thrilling, but not always pleasant. I like to get ahead of the curve and surf. And, knowing my destiny is inextricably linked to my community, I like to build arks, not just surfboards. Call the 10-mile diet prototyping arks.

There is no special virtue in a 10-mile diet. Or a 50-mile or 100-mile diet. The miles are simply markers for something else: bringing our eating closer to home. Why? We have lost touch with "the hands that feed us" to our detriment, and this story is meant to show you what's at the other end of the industrial food scale, to help you see that there are reasonable and heartening alternatives.

This book, then, is not about pious restraint. It is not about sucking it up and making do. It's a banquet of good stories and possible skillful interventions that can tilt us toward food sufficiency. I describe the hows and whys of my 10-mile diet experiment, what I discovered, what I loved, what I hated, what I missed, what I learned, and a level of body and soul satisfaction I barely knew existed. It was only a month of that extreme, but they say new habits take twenty-one days to anchor, and so it was for me.

The 10-mile diet changed me. I blogged every day, diving into food issues, awakening sleeping-beauty skills of cooking and gardening and reengaging with an old passion for social change, sidelined while I recovered from cancer. Best of all, I finally landed somewhere on earth, in a real place with real soil and forests, a real community where I belong the way my skin belongs to me. I am part of life; not at a remove in self-sufficiency but connected in reciprocity, mutuality, and care.

Whidbey was a perfect place to run this experiment. In fact, if I lived across Puget Sound in Seattle, a 10-mile diet would have been far harder. Even with all the backyard gardens there, it's mostly paved and built up. When I lived there, I always had a patch of lettuce and kale in the yard, but little about Seattle says, "Eat here," so a 10-mile diet might not even have occurred to me. The point, though, isn't for you to replicate what I did. I scouted out a possibility and documented it here because it points at a way out of our dependency on the centralized, industrial scale food system. As you will see, when you look at a broader definition of local food, we can all provision ourselves regionally—if we commit to personal and political change.

I begin the book by telling the story of who I was when I took up the 10-mile diet challenge, including the worldview that primed me to want to do it and the scramble to find the hands that grew the food that would feed me that month. You will meet Tricia, the market gardener who grew most of the food I ate, as well as other gardeners, farmers, and ranchers. Then you will follow, week by week, the ups and downs of my 10-mile month. After it's over, I'll evaluate the experiment, mine the gold. You will also join me on a hunt for answers to the question How dependent are we and do we need to be on the industrial food system to feed ourselves and the world? My tale ends with some key ideas about what weights we can put on the local side of the scale to give regional food systems a larger role in nourishing us all. I refer to these flourishing local food landscapes as "complementary food systems," not supplanting the global supply chains but expanding consumer food choice. The goal, of course, is fair, affordable, accessible, healthy, delicious, and nourishing food for all. Who could disagree?

You will develop a new sense about feeding yourself, which I call "relational eating." It is the shift from being a lone eater in the endless food courts of the industrial system, treating the hands that feed you like vending machines, to standing in the middle of your food system, with nourishment all around in the gardens, fields, farms, forests, and waters of your region. You are in relationship with these ever-widening circles of food, from daily habits to windowsill sprouts to backyard vegetable plots to neighborhood farm stands and gardens to the stores, CSA (community supported agriculture) membership farms, farmers' markets, and more in your community, your regional food sheds, and beyond.

I make no effort to be definitive, exhaustive, or authoritative. If I waited for *that,* I'd never give you my mostly baked notions for your investigation. Also, local food is a passion and practice in rapid cultural ascendancy. A book cannot contain all there is to know as the field is changing daily. I'm sure that people in the know will challenge or correct me and that many of my readers have their own stories to tell and expertise to share. Being part of a rising tide of knowledge in the making is part of what makes local food so delicious. We're in this together.

Hope

This is not just a story of food, though. It is a story of rekindling hope at a time when positive change seems harder than ever, when solving our global energy, economic, and environmental issues fairly and squarely seems almost impossible despite how much our politicians try to cheer us up with promises.

I'm a boomer. Those of us who chose to use our postwar birthright of opportunity to change the world made great strides in justice, fairness, environmental protection, and cultural transformation. I and my personal team (the New Road Map Foundation) set ourselves the wee goal of ending overconsumption in North America, of teaching, supporting, and even cajoling people to live within their means. By the end of the last millennium I had to admit that despite writing a best seller, despite the tens of thousands of people who say *Your Money or Your Life* changed their lives, we had failed to reach the larger goal we'd set: that Americans would collectively and voluntarily resize our consumption to what the earth can sustainably provide.

Coming out of my cancer years, the only hope I could see was adaptation to the consequences of inaction and ignorance: a diminished and changing earth. I found the relocalization movement and a pinhole of hope opened. But the 10-mile diet set off a gusher of natural hope, a confidence that the conditions for thriving and resilience are all around us and that food—revitalizing regional food systems—is a collective project worthy of our best efforts.

Is Local for You?

Local uniquely connects you, an eater, with the hands that feed you—your farmer, the food s/he cultivates and harvests, and the place you both live. Every one of us has this opportunity to reinhabit the land that nurtures us—that gives us life.

Before we began to "eat" fossil fuel—before this concentrated energy source changed everything about what and how we eat—most of us were involved in home production—whether growing or preserving or preparing from scratch our daily fare. Two hundred years ago in the United States, local was the way everyone ate, and farming was the primary profession—90 percent of Americans lived on farms. "Takeout"—eating food from nowhere, cooked by people you don't know, put in Styrofoam to eat at home, possibly alone—is not the way any of us had been raised—until now! As much of a miracle as this disconnected way of eating is for busy people who want to do and make and influence more than dinner, we need to acknowledge that it has literally ungrounded us.

Making some small commitment to eating within a radius of where you live is an act of reconnection. It is an act of honoring the hands and lands that feed you. Food becomes where you live and who you live with, not just another consumer item. Thus eating local food becomes ethical and spiritual as well as all the other reasons to do it—sociability of farmers' markets, freshness, unique and diverse cultivars, greater nutrition.

Local also matters in a larger context. Our apparently lush food system is like a giant flower on a spindly stalk. Look at the flower and everything is beautiful and right. Peer underneath at the stalk and you realize how precarious it is. You enjoy the bounty—yet every day you wonder when it will snap. The system itself assures us that nothing is wrong. But we now know that every aspect of that beautiful flower depends on fossil fuel not just to transport crisp apples from New Zealand or grapes from Chile but to fertilize those distant soils and protect those faraway plants from pests and even support the rapid prototyping of new hybrid seeds. New technologies may let us extract more oil now than before, but the basic supply is finite. That voluptuous dahlia of the fresh food section at your Whole Foods market is like a painted curtain or a projected image—real enough, but not really real for really long.

I will introduce you to what *is real* to me—the interesting and informative farmers and gardeners and chefs and institutions of Whidbey Island in the far Northwest of the United States. Meeting them you will see how local works in reality, and the extraordinary joys as well as challenges of rehabilitating local food systems.

Will Local Make You Thin, Rich, Healthy, and Eternal?

Let's get this self-help promise over with. Half a century of relentless advertising and half a millennium (at least) of fire-and-brimstone religion have stoked our darkest fears of being cast out, lonely, sick, rejected, unloved, and vulnerable. We'd buy anything that could save us from that fate, which is truly worse than death.

The self-help industry thrives on these fears and offers personal salvation. Let's see how local measures up.

Want to Get Thin?

Once you participate in growing food or at least in the lives of the farmers who grow your food, you are less likely to waste it.

Industrial food is easy and cheap and loaded with sugar and fat. The "business" of food is profit, so we, the eaters, are cajoled, exhorted, and enticed to eat too much, broadening our bottoms as we feed the corporate bottom line. And food in the United States is surprisingly cheap; no people on earth spend as little as we do on food as a percentage of our budget. This means that we have few speed bumps on our highway to overeating.

On my 10-mile diet I lost six pounds in a month, partly because I ate no grain, but also because I ate with reverence and respect for my "feeders."

Want to Get Healthy?

Unless you live next to a megafarm, feed lot, or some food-processing plant where one or more of the hundreds of nonfood ingredients found in many food products get added, local food means simpler, more basic, and less toxic food. While this is not a screed against manufactured food, it is an invitation to rethink what, beyond real food, goes into your body and whether those additives are truly necessary for food to be delicious and easy to prepare. I loved the rich, flavorful food I ate in my 10-mile month—and beyond. I had energy all day long—and my bad cholesterol went down and good cholesterol went up.

Want More Money?

Even though local food is often more expensive—sometimes far more expensive—than manufactured food, you get some of that money back through the nutritional value. According to the *Journal of the*

Science of Food and Agriculture, the high heat of canning causes some loss of vitamins C and B.[1] And, as you will learn, industrial agriculture is like the Red Queen and locally produced food is like Alice. The rules change often and immediately to favor the imperious monarch. The playing field isn't level or even a gentle slant. Local producers have to huff and puff up some very steep hills of regulations and just can't compete on industrial agriculture's terms. It's not up to you and me to make up for all that, to spend more in service to our local growers, but it is up to all of us to participate in some way in changing the rules enough to make farming viable for young and new farmers. Currently less than 2 percent of our population farms. The average age of farmers is close to sixty. We needed a generation of scientists for technological prowess in the era of Sputnik and beyond. We now need a generation of farmers in order to eat well into the future.

Want to Live Forever?

No one can give you that. Religion may promise you an afterlife, which could be quite appealing if you are suffering in this one, but there is no tangible proof of it. Here's what local food can promise in that domain. Love. You are supporting your neighbors—and they are feeding you. You are weaving your community together in the most basic way. You are rewarding the hard work of those who farm in some measure by hand. The industrial food system of my youth, just when it was flexing its muscles, promised that your food was "untouched by human hands." For our families in the fifties, disconnection was white bread was love. Local food *is* touched by human hands and that is the point. You are loving and serving the hands that feed you. Love, according to all religion, is the highest value. And who knows, that may get you into heaven.

Thriving Together

Local eating could seem like a personal choice that only hippies or Yuppies might make, but it is actually a collective project for a shared future. How to do that is the question. How do we have our (local) cake and eat it too (not sacrifice the benefits of anywhere food)? This is the challenge. By what agreements, compromises, laws, customs, rituals, or celebrations will we bring forth on this earth a future of common resilience, flourishing together?

In the seventies when we were waking up to spirituality, we'd say "the longest journey is the twelve inches between head and heart." Now the necessary journey is "from me to we," from self-interest to common interest, from YOYO (you're on your own) to WAITT (slow down, we're all in this together). The task now is to gather up our hard-earned freedoms and apply them to shaping a future that works for all. As it says in the Bible in Matthew 5:45, "He makes his sun to rise on the evil and on the good, and sends rain on the just and on the unjust." Same with the earth's living systems—what affects them affects us all. The sun and rain of climate change fall on everyone. No one has the option of cutting loose from the collective, presuming she can make it on her own or survive at the expense of others.

We need to find a way to be free—and cooperate. To be creative and work for the common good. In short, to be part of a community and to be fully ourselves. What I call relational eating—being in relationship with the food, farms, farmers, forests, waters, soils, air, and other critters in a local living food system—is such a path.

The Age of Resilience

I believe we are in a new age, the age of resilience—the capacity to roll with the punches. Smart people in the age of resilience are resourceful—able to make the most of what's at hand. Relocalization is bringing more of what we need closer to our hands. Fear, though, will weaken both resilience and resourcefulness. I want to inspire you to live this adventure, to whatever degree you choose, with me and all of us in these times. I want to be inspired and motivated by *your* creativity and heart. Research shows that people rise to the occasion when they must—they muster courage and help one another and offer solace in the face of loss. What's ahead is an occasion we will all rise to—and we'll all do it right where we are: on islands, like me; in forgotten rural communities; in suburbs and cities. There is hope everywhere. Even in regions around the world impoverished for a host of reasons, communities are taking control of their destiny, re-localizing.

This, then, is where the 10-mile diet landed me. I could easily go back to old habits, but I haven't. I am aware of where my food comes from. I buy from my neighbors if at all possible, buy from my region as much as I can, and buy fair trade for food pleasures from afar if I can. I also buy those foods I love that come from everywhere/nowhere—and there are plenty of them. I'm transformed but not reborn. I simply like being acquainted with my food. I like cooking from scratch. I like eating less with more gratitude. I like growing what I can. I like being part of a global conversation about local eating—and adding my spice to the stew. I like the political puzzle—which policy shifts and personal choices and skillful practices will rebalance our food system. I like being part of this unfolding story, the shared adventure in security, sovereignty, and safety; in health, prosperity, and yum. And I like being relaxed about it all.

Food is our primary form of consumption. Transforming our relationship with food and the hands that feed us transforms so much else. I invite you to sit down at this banquet of stories and new ideas and nibble and graze and chew and digest and see how it all goes down. I invite you to simply enjoy yourself. If you find things you want to try, do so in a spirit of curiosity and good cheer. At the end of each chapter, a section called "Now It's Your Turn" offers some action steps that, once you've read the whole book, you can come back to and try out. Between chapters are some wonderful recipes using regional ingredients from the creative kitchens of fine local chefs, assembled by the star chef in the book, Jess Dowdell. There's something for everyone to savor—the gourmet, the activist, the lover of good tales. Bon appétit!

CHAPTER ONE

Localize Me?

~~~~~~~~~

July 4, 2010

The sun was warm, the sky clear, and, frankly, hyperlocal eating was nowhere on my radar. My only interest in eating locally was grabbing a bite of some German potato salad gracing the banquet table—dead ahead—laden with potluck dishes. Yet amazingly, I was about to sign on to an experiment in 10-mile eating that would redirect my life. Join me in my final hour of "anywhere eating."

Let me set the scene. My clan of friends had come out of their home offices and back from their travels to celebrate the Fourth of July at our annual potluck picnic near Maxwelton Beach, one of the original settlements on the western shore of South Whidbey Island. Soon we would, with heaping plates of food, watch the funky-to-the-max Maxwelton Parade: the classic cars and political protest floats and whale puppets and waving political candidates and belly dancers and children wearing gossamer wings—all of whom promenade at two miles per hour along the dead-end beach road, throwing candy at us gawkers. We'd ooh and aah and eat and socialize and relax and watch the sun set behind the Olympic Mountains across Useless Bay.

Two hundred years ago, had you looked out over that very stretch of beach, you might have seen Lower Skagit First Nations people feasting on salmon, deer, perhaps duck supplemented with nettles and camas roots. A hundred years ago the Salish would have been gone and you occasionally might have seen thousands of people from all around the region gathered for a Chautauqua, a two-week festival of entertainment, edification, and inspiration. They would have carried picnic baskets filled with eggs and garden vegetables and meats and pies, almost all of it local food. People from miles around came to the five-thousand-seat amphitheater, built with the abundant lumber on the island by the first settlers, the Mackies, who'd arrived in 1905 on a steamboat, barging all their possessions ashore except for their milk cow Bossy . . . who swam.

Now here we all were, transplants to this island, many of us earning money off the island as consultants, writers, knowledge workers, and retirees, enabling us to live the good life here. Ahead of us were tables filled with dishes from every part of the planet: teriyaki chicken wings and hand-rolled sushi from Japan, fried rice from China, tabbouleh salad from the Middle East, potato salad from South America, chutneys from India, pasta from Italy, potato latkes from Poland. All of them considered American foods now.

The green salads alone were the world in a bowl. Lettuce from the Central Valley in California, cucumbers from China, tomatoes from Mexico, avocados from the tropics, salad oil from Venezuela, vinegar from China, pepper from Vietnam, and salt from the Himalayas. The sugar in the desserts was probably from Brazil.

I was a pretty sick puppy when I transplanted myself to this island in Puget Sound five years earlier. After decades of "saving the world" it seemed the thing I actually needed to save was my own life. I was diagnosed in 2004 with stage-three colon cancer. Strangely, the news seemed less like a verdict and more like a hall pass from carrying the world on my back as if I were the sole refueling ship on the way to the space station and the stars. It might have been the surgery that saved my life. It might have been the bit of chemotherapy I received that proved so vile I quit. It might have been, though, that I faced myself and changed my life—and I was officially well, though exhausted. That's when I came to this motherly island, and was brought back to full vitality by the very waters and mountains across the way and by the very people on that potluck line. I was healthy, I was happy, and I was ready to jump into life again.

I was also a lot lighter—not from the chemo but from a six-week marathon diet that had stripped twenty pounds off my body and promised to have changed my metabolism so that I could now eat gloriously, wantonly, voluptuously, without ever gaining back a pound. Having paid my dues, the payoff was this very meal, these glistening dishes full of fat and sugar and salt, crunch and slither and squish, noodles and rice and everything nice that I'd been denied trying to regain my menopause-obliterated waist.

I was trying not to look too eager as I clutched my plate and eyed the spread ahead with all the casualness of a hungry dog when he's about to get fed. I flicked my tongue to both corners of my mouth, in case I was drooling.

Until this day, the only "food issues" that got my attention were personal. They were all about feeding my mouth, not feeding the world. In two decades of writing and teaching about the perils of overconsumption, I had challenged only our obsession with money and things and their impact on the planet, not our obsession with food, eating and dieting. How could I challenge our food insanity when I had my own hand in the cookie jar?

How Have I Dieted? Let Me Count the Ways

I'd always been an eater, of course. I was born that way. The simple act of bending my elbow with food-laden forks and spoons would amount, over my lifetime, to more than six tons of food disappearing down my gullet. What I have to show for all that shoveling is that I'm alive . . . with a few extra pounds.

The first time the bliss of feeding turned to the shame of fat was when I was six. On a hot day at a summer camp far more progressive than my parents knew, we were invited to take off our shirts and run in the sun. I watched kids with rail-thin bodies and ribs like keyboards tear their shirts off. I was pudgy—and mortified. In those days I loved cinch belts, so I valiantly hiked mine up from waist to underarms like a tube top and wiggled my hips like a movie actress, smiled, and came to know that I was different. I was fat.

The cinch belt was, in fact, the first of many elastic strategies for shaving off the odd bump and lump. "We've got to get you into a girdle," my mother hissed one day as she walked behind me and saw that puberty was rearranging my fat attractively into two round dancing butt cheeks. We went directly to B. Altman's foundations department to sausage me into a body shaper that could second as a chastity belt. Sometime later our family physician put me on my first diet. He had a big, sloppy, tobacco-stained gray mustache and his own balloon of a belly and delivered a sheet of paper with "the diet" with the same authority as God handing those two tablets to Moses. Dry toast. Skim milk. Naked vegetables. Sliced fruit. Skinless chicken.

So began a lifetime of diets and cheating on diets. I replaced pleasure and appetite with lists of dos and don'ts—and more diets than beads on a rosary. From Atkins to Fat Flush to Zone to South Beach to raw food to no food (fasting) so I could remember what my ribs and hip bones felt like—but, like the tide, the fat rolled in again and I rolled my self into a girdle as a last resort.

Then there were the health and virtue diets. Eat no fish (fisheries are collapsing). Eat no red meat (bad for your arteries and definitely bad for the feedlot cows). Eat no chicken (mass-produced in cages). Eat no dairy—you're probably allergic. Eat no eggs—cholesterol. No, wait, eat eggs, you need the lecithin. Eat nothing with eyes (our brothers and sisters)—only fruits, nuts, and vegetables. When I lived in the woods in northern Wisconsin, tending a half-acre garden with a group of friends, we took a photo of us brandishing guns and knives at a wheelbarrow full of fresh-killed vegetables—yanked from the ground and piled high like carcasses. I dabbled in food virtue, one "right way" after another—and went back to eating what I wanted, working only on the virtue of self-acceptance.

The derivation of *diet* from the Greek means simply "how you live." Traditionally it simply meant what people eat; cultures identify with the foods of their land—the salmon people, the seal people, the reindeer people, the taro people. Are we, then, the fast-food people? The aspartame people? Have we lost our "diet"—our way of life— entirely in service to dieting? If you review the many diets,[1] few agree what to limit. Ayurvedic practitioners even question the supremacy of chugging down eight glasses of water a day. We should sip, not gulp. It should be warm, not cold.

I even lost any honest hunger, that inbred signal to get up and seek food. Hunger was always an option, welcome because it meant my diet was working; my body was finally eating its stores of fat. In my whole life I might have missed meals, but I've never gone hungry involuntarily for more than a day. My hungers were for things food could not really solve—because I was sad or scared or frustrated or bored. I bit down on food so I wouldn't snap at the next person to cross my path.

Am I the only one this nuts? I don't think so. We treat our bodies like servants or mannequins or machines or sex objects or conveyances for our overactive brains—rarely as a simple blessing, an aliveness. Food thus becomes a temptation, the enemy, a pleasure money can buy, an ostentation, a trifle, a given. Many of us have a love-hate relationship with food. We binge. We purge. We won't eat. We won't stop eating. If news of hunger and starvation wafts in on the morning news as we drink our fruit smoothie or eat sausage and eggs, at best we write a check—and perhaps later in the day assuage our uneasy conscience by another visit to the fridge.

How perfect that I was about to begin the 10-mile diet just as I'd finished feeding my fat-hating demon one more time. No longer a little girl at summer camp who could hike up a cinch belt to fit in, I was inching, literally, toward a matronly body—and I didn't like it. That's why I joined a growing number of friends in using a new super diet—the standard starvation plus a hormone that aids weight loss the way steroids aid muscle bulk. They'd all lost upward twenty pounds. Now I had too and was about to celebrate my win . . . by eating.

I did not know what I was in for with the 10-mile diet. I never expected to develop a new relationship with food that had nothing—but nothing—to do with my size. I would fall in love with the hands and lands that fed me. I would learn to seek nourishment, connection, and empowerment through how I grew, bought, cooked, and ate my food. I, the lone eater, would become I, the blessed, with food, farmers, farms, fields, and forests that fed me. I would receive the love right from the food, rather than turning to food as a substitute for love. This kind of diet sticks because it transforms the eater.

Local food could be yet one more fad or one more issue or one more virtue. Something to try—and say you did. The experiment I would soon undertake required an honest look at my current relationship with food. How I used food as an emotional crutch, as a ritual, as an entitlement, as an identity, as a set of habits I had no desire to break. On that summer day in 2010, though, local food was simply the happy distance between plate and mouth.

Growing Up in the Fifties

Most of us at the potluck had grown up in the fertile soil of the post–World War II middle class. We grew up hearing:

"Eat your vegetables. Think of the poor starving children in . . . [China, Korea, Africa]."

"Don't ruin your appetite." (Which meant no snacking after four P.M. Ruining our appetites was a sin against Mother, who spent an hour cooking our dinner.)

"If you don't eat your dinner you can't have any dessert."

"Clean Plate Club!"

Our parents were reflecting their experience during the Depression, when so many did not have enough to eat. Meager fare continued into the war effort. Until the year I was born, sugar, coffee, processed foods, meats, canned fish, cheese, canned milk, and fats were all rationed, and victory gardens fed the nation.

After all that privation, the United States liked its women rounder. Marilyn Monroe was a size 14, compared to the size 6 stars of today. We weren't afraid of a little weight. Milkmen delivered creamy fresh milk in glass bottles—plus butter and eggs—to the rising middle class's doors daily. Fear of the link between high cholesterol and heart disease was still in the future. Elsie wasn't yet a cartoon character standing on hind legs, a frilly apron around her waist. No, Elsie was a real cow and she lived, like I did, on Long Island. And we put big dollops of real butter on our hot vegetables before serving them.

Food miles back then weren't an issue because most food was at least regional. Sure, we had Wonder bread from the breadbasket of the nation and the new frozen, canned, and boxed foods made elsewhere. But the hundreds of additives we now ingest were still gleams in chemists' eyes.

My first foray from the confines of home was to that progressive camp in Tenants Harbor, Maine, where we had Lobster Feast Day each year. We each got a whole one-dollar fresh-caught lobster to drown in butter and eat with bibs that never kept us clean. We'd cook the lobsters in giant black-bottomed stockpots over a fire on the beach, plunging them in boiling water and then piling seaweed on top to steam our now bright-red lobsters to perfect rubbery doneness. The cook also harvested a lacy white seaweed and made seaweed pudding that I bragged about to playmates stuck on Long Island.

"I ate seaweed."

"Yuk."

"A lot you know. It was really good."

Later I went farther, tasted more. Every winter the family migrated to Hollywood Beach, Florida. Our three-day drives from Hempstead, Long Island, were punctuated by stops at Stuckey's, the old pecan and tchotchkes shops along the great American highways of the fifties. You always knew how far the next Stuckey's was. As soon as you drove out of one there was the billboard: ONLY 247 MILES TO THE NEXT STUCKEY'S. My brother and I kept track of Stuckey's distances like gamblers keep track of the odds.

Coming of Age in the Sixties

My food circles widened as the years went on. Opportunities to indulge my insatiable curiosity kept coming as I went farther afield.

In Austria I sampled fresh yogurt. In Spain I ate *calamares en su tinta* (squid in its own ink) and *morcillo* (blood sausage) and *tortillas,* which there meant frittatas of potatoes and onions cooked in olive oil. In Norway I ate goat cheese and lutefisk, drank aquavit, and sang "Tak für Matten" before the meal. In Russia I gorged on black caviar. Intourist, the Soviet tourism bureaucracy, required visitors to purchase meal tickets in advance—enough for caviar and chicken Kiev for breakfast, lunch, and dinner. In Mexico I learned to hunt turtle eggs in the early morning on the beach and to grind potent chiles, salt, and garlic in a stone molcajete for killer hot sauce. My neighbors—literally barefoot and pregnant—taught me to slap masa between my hands into thick Mexican tortillas and cook them over a wood fire. In Cuba I ate greasy arroz con pollo, fried plantains, and moros y cristianos (black beans and rice). In Thailand I ate sticky rice. In Hungary I actually had goulash. I fasted in the desert and gorged at the King's Table in Las Vegas. I ate around. And unto roundness.

In a way, coming to Whidbey Island in 2005 after fifteen years of globetrotting was coming down to earth again. It could well be that the chicken in the bubbling Crock-Pot on the potluck table had roamed free in one of my neighbors' yards and been beheaded, bled, gutted, and plucked by the very hands now giving a final stir to the fragrant stew.

Within an hour, I'd agree to start my road back to eating where I am planted, but for another few minutes the world of anywhere eating was my oyster—and whatever else on that table I could get onto my plate. It didn't seem unreasonable that in addition to some home-grown salads there were three kinds of corn chips and five kinds of salsa. Nor did it seem strange to me that flavors from India and Africa were combined in one rice dish or fruits from three continents were in a fruit salad. The exotic has almost become humdrum to us.

By now I had snagged a piece of pie just to be sure and was beginning to scoop small mounds of each appealing dish onto my plate, tightly arranged from the center out like packed sunflower seeds in mature, laden heads. I was maximizing the plate. I would give a new meaning to "super-size me."

Overeating

Overeating is as American as apple pie. We are free to consume as much as we want whenever we want—and no one can stop us. Corporate food companies advertise on TV and on the Internet and in the pages of magazines and on roadside billboards knowing that as we gain, they gain. They pack us as full as possible—like geese bred for foie gras—and tell us this is freedom and choice and happiness. It all tastes so good that we comply, not realizing how scientific the manipulation of taste is. Our palates evolved in nature, where sugar and fat are rare and rich sources of energy, and salts contain precious minerals. In the presence of any of these, our brains flash Go, assuming such rich fare is limited. A stop signal wasn't needed.

But now we aren't hunters in the wild, we are consumers in the endless food courts of the early third millennium—global eaters with reptilian brains. Products laden with fat, sugar, and salt—or all three (salted caramel ice cream, anyone?) are readily available in fast-food drive-throughs and full refrigerators everywhere. In a stroke of evolutionary brilliance, Frito-Lay nailed it when they advertised "Bet you can't eat just one."

I filled my plate as if I, like my ancestors, didn't know when a feast like this would come my way again. We do know, though. Probably in three hours. But hardwired habits are hard to shake. Finally liberated from the constraint of the strict diet I'd been on, I was doing what comes naturally—getting ready to gorge. Could it be that I wouldn't just expand back into my old two-size-larger clothes after the extreme diet? The diet's originator promised otherwise. I chose to believe him. To imagine I was not only two sizes smaller but had the metabolism of a teenage jock.

I wandered out to engage in the happy ritual of drifting from one group to another, renewing acquaintances, meeting new people, hearing about births, deaths, marriages, divorces, and the migrations of children off the island and back on. We talked politics but without too much passion, and about personal trials without too much detail.

Content didn't matter much. We were just happy little bees rubbing antennae.

The 10-Mile Diet Begins

As I was enjoying the infinite pleasures of eating in good company, Tricia Beckner wandered by with her husband, Kent Ratekin. Tricia has short, highlighted hair that she ruffles as if to punctuate her sentences. We officially met as sopranos in the Open Circle Singers, a no-audition choir that let me actually sing instead of—as I had been instructed in school—just move my lips in sync with the tuneful. I'd joined the choir the first month I was here, discovered I hit more notes dead-on as a soprano, and found myself next to Tricia weekly, mumbling jokes between songs.

I'd seen her, actually, in another setting that I hoped she did not remember. My new apartment came with a garden plot and I needed some manure to enrich the soil before planting. A normal person would have bought a bag of precomposted steer manure, but not frugal me, not with sheep next door. Indeed, that paddock had dung galore—on the other side of a fence. I waited till dusk, climbed the fence, and started to fill my bucket. A car had passed by, and even though I crouched at the sound, Tricia (the driver) told me later that she'd noted a strange sight of someone apparently—could it be?—stealing poop.

But Tricia wasn't thinking about manure bandits when she saw me. She had something else on her mind. "Hey," she said, "Kent and I were watching this thing on YouTube last night. You know Morgan Spurlock? *Super Size Me?*"

I only nodded because my tongue was now squishing creamy Yellow Finn potato salad onto the roof of my mouth.

"Yeah, well, I saw this Netflix movie where this guy did a 'super-high me' thing. Smoked pot every day for a month. So I said to Kent, 'You should do a "super-veggie me." Eat only what grows in my garden for thirty days. Sort of a reverse *Super Size Me.*'" Tricia has a half-acre garden where she grows both for home use and for sale from a stand by the Langley post office. "He said no."

"Are *you* going to try it?"

"Heck no. No way I could do that. I can't live without my treats. But I decided to see if someone else would. I've asked a dozen people so far and no one is game. It's probably impossible."

"I'll do it," I said, shifting from the German potato salad to a cherry pie so sweet I am sure the main ingredients were white sugar followed by cornstarch, with some cherries mixed in to merit being called cherry pie.

Sustainability as Extreme Sport

Lifestyle experiments are like extreme sports for me. As soon as I had language I'd try new things and run to Mother saying, "You know something?" and give a report on my latest discovery. In the years since, I've lived in an operatic range of temperatures—from the coldest (Rhinelander, Wisconsin) to the hottest (Florence, Arizona) parts of the country. I lived for years in a motor home with just forty cubic feet to call my own: thirty-five cubic feet for sleeping, five cubic feet for possessions. For six years I lived on one hundred dollars a month. I hiked solo in the Anza Borrego Desert, fasting for three days in a cave by a huge rock clearly used by the aboriginals for grinding seeds and corn into a powder with a stone. None of this felt like suffering or deprivation or even risk. It felt like going to the edge of the known to see what I—and the world—was made of. Live for a month on what Tricia grows in her garden for farmers' market sales? Sure. Not just sure, but "Hell yes! Bring it on!"

And so it was that I undertook hyperlocal eating with no other expertise than being an eater who by now had packed away much of my lifetime tonnage of food to relieve stress, to taste the world, to celebrate and mourn, to tap out the rhythms of my days.

I wasn't a foodie. I was lapsed from every diet—political, weight loss, or spiritual—I'd ever tried. My story may have a few more twists, turns, and wrinkles than yours, but we all have a food history and food psychology and food values. We each have a relationship with food that isn't necessarily right or wrong, good or bad, but simply part of the narrative of our lives. This history steers our behavior no matter what high-minded course we set ourselves on.

The challenge made so casually at a potluck was going to put me on the road to learning more about myself than just how to cook a turnip.

Now It's Your Turn

Do you want to delve into your own relationship with food? Here are some questions and exercises to guide you. This is not a quick women's magazine self-test. The questions and suggestions will worm their way into you. Your answers may change over time. You don't need to stop reading until you finish all these exercises! Read through the questions and exercises, digest them, and read on. Chapter 2 is where you will see why, once I'd said yes, I was dead serious about going local.

Who are you as an eater? To look at yourself as an eater (not a dieter!), here are some questions:

- What does food mean to you—fuel, love, comfort, chore, pleasure?
- What are your "must have" foods, and why must you have them?
- Why might you have said "Hell no" or "Hell yes" if Tricia had proposed to you a radical experiment in local eating?
- Where do your food preferences come from—your family, your culture, your travels, your values, your feelings about your body, your emotional states?
- What are your guilty pleasures? Your must-have food necessities?
- Are these preferences anywhere near your values? Your sense of fairness and justice? Your faith and politics? Your need to slow down and smell the snow peas?

Your Life as an Eater

To help you dig into your life as an eater, here are some prompts to uncork memories:

- What did I eat as a child?
- Who cooked for me? Did they teach me to cook?
- What were my family meals like? Did we actually eat together? Did we watch TV or converse or, today, text?
- What are my favorite foods and why do I like them?
- What did I eat at family holidays? My wedding? In the school cafeteria?
- Did my parents or grandparents or even great-grandparents tell me anything about food when they were young? My mother grew up in New York City; the iceman was a daily feature of life, and earlier still the fishmongers came through.
- What new foods did I encounter as I grew up—and where?
- When did I first get to choose what I ate?
- Was food used for rewards and punishments? Was it associated with pleasure? Pain? Guilt? Rebellion?
- Did I change what I ate when I changed my social group, took a new job, lived somewhere new?
- What were my family's food rules—their dos and don'ts? How has that affected me?
- And how did I feel about it all—the food, the meals, the cooking?

Your Life as a Dieter

If you have altered your eating to lose weight, gain health, get closer to heaven, or live your ethics, you can go down that memory lane.

TELL YOUR FOOD STORIES

Weave these memories into the story of your life.

MAKE A FOOD TIME LINE

Draw a line, with one end your birth and the other today. Divide it into years or decades or life's seasons (child, teen, young adult, etc.). Write memories along the time line, like "Mom's grilled cheese sandwiches" or

"Using the wrong fork at a formal dinner" or "White Tower burgers" or "Buying fish right from a boat in San Francisco." Include the food trends and fads that came and went in your life, and extend your time line back before you were born. What were the foods of your parents, grandparents, and great-grandparents? These are the people who formed you as an eater.

WRITE ABOUT A MEMORY

Use as a writing prompt one of the memories that evoke strong feelings—nostalgia, fear, happiness, friendship, domination, guilt. See what story pops out of "grilled cheese" or "the right fork" or "when my mother . . ." Make the story vivid and detailed. Where were you? Who was there and how did you feel about each person. Was it an ordinary day or a special occasion? Include what people were wearing, the sound of their voices, how the air in the room felt, the smells and tastes. What happened as the incident unfolded? Is it a story of comfort, of conflict, of a change in your life, of your crazy family, or what? Read the story aloud to a friend—having a witness is inherently moving.

HAVE A FOOD CONVERSATION

Through writing my blog and now this book I've discovered that everyone has a food story—and they love to tell it. Introduce the topic at a family meal or reunion, or over coffee with a friend. Host a potluck with everyone bringing a food from their youth and talking about it. Start a blog or a Facebook page and invite people to tell their stories.

MAKE A COLLAGE

Even people who think they can't draw or compose music can use the art of others for collage—a powerful way to explore the soul of your relationship with food. Just get a stack of magazines and leaf through them, tearing out pictures that appeal to you without questioning why you are attracted to each one. Get out a piece of paper or cardboard and a glue stick. Pick from your collection—letting your unconscious speak—

the pictures or fragments of pictures you want, trim them as you like (you may just pick a detail, a hand with a ring, a cherry), place them on the paper, and when you have an arrangement that speaks to you, glue them down. It's pretty amazing to do this quietly with a group of people and then tell the story of your collage.

WHAT ARE YOUR FOOD MESSAGES?

Food messages are the instructions we absorb from family, culture, religion, society, and friends about how, what, why, when, and with whom to eat. They are the commandments, the dos and don'ts, the rights and wrongs, the goods and bads, of food. You may not even be aware of them, which is why identifying them can be so liberating. Some food messages are quite useful, and some are more toxic than the mystery ingredients in processed food.

- There are rules about when to eat—three squares a day; not after nine P.M.; only when you are truly hungry.
- There are rules about what to eat—no red meat; nothing with eyes; no animal products; no wheat; nothing cooked.
- There are rules about where to eat—not in your car; not standing up at the kitchen counter.
- There are rules about whom to eat with—daily family meals; never eat alone; eat in silence, attending to every bite.
- There are cultural rules about how to eat—don't smack your lips; yes, smack your lips; don't belch; yes, belch; not with your hands; only with your hands.
- There are the diet gurus, from Oz to Ornish to Atkins, who dish up their rules with absolute certainty.

What food messages have you internalized? What foods do you label "good" and "bad" and why? Make a short list.

This is just the beginning of your engagement as a relational eater—which is what I became thanks to the adventure you'll read about in the coming chapters.

Try These Recipes

Jess Dowdell, whom you will meet in chapter 7, is now proprietress of the Roaming Radish, a deli, catering, and cooking class establishment. Passionate about local food and cooking, she can rattle off where she gets every ingredient, and who grew the greens or raised the lamb or roasted the coffee. When I wanted to include recipes in this book, I turned to her to know which chefs and farmers to approach and where to place each recipe in the narrative. Since I began this 10-mile diet journey at a potluck, here are two recipes from Jess for picnic-type foods.

Local Bean Hummus

2 cups dried Rockwell beans
½ cup chopped parsley
1 jalapeño pepper, minced
1 tablespoon honey
¼ cup minced garlic
¼ cup lemon juice
Salt and pepper to taste

Soak the beans for 12 hours, then cook them in a large pot over medium heat until they are soft. Drain and rinse them in cold water. When the beans are cool, transfer to a blender or food processor and blend them with the parsley, jalapeño, honey, garlic, and lemon juice. Add salt and pepper to taste. Add a little oil if needed to get a nice pureed-hummus consistency.

Bread and Butter Pickles

10 local pickling cucumbers (Patty and Loren from Quail's Run grow
the best!)
1 cup salt

Slice the cucumbers to the desired size, then mix with the salt and 3
pounds of ice, cover with water, press the cucumber slices down with a
weighted lid, and let sit for 3 hours. Rinse the cucumbers and set them
aside.

In a large stock pot bring the following ingredients to a boil:

3 cups apple cider vinegar
3 cups sugar
½ cup mustard seeds
¼ cup coriander
¼ cup dill seed
2 tablespoons turmeric

When the sugar is dissolved, add the cucumber slices and bring the water back to a boil. As soon as it boils you are done. Pack the pickles in jars
to can or let them cool and store in your fridge.

Sweet Pickle Relish

Take 2 cups of your bread and butter pickles and 1 onion and chop
them together. Great on burgers!

CHAPTER TWO

Putting My Mouth Where My Mouth Is

Holy (local) cow! I thought when I got home. Can I actually survive for a month just on what Tricia grows? Go meatless and fatless and sugarless for thirty days? What have I signed up for?

I'd agreed in part because the challenge was my kind of quirky, but also because I'd already signed up for the bigger game: lowering consumption here in the United States because of the damage we're doing to the earth—and our souls. Besides, I was no stranger to do-it-yourself and grow-your-own. Even though I'd gone soft since settling down, exercising my mind while my butt spread in my swivel/recline/snooze office chair, earlier in my life I'd lived one of the standard story lines of my generation: go on the road (thank you, Ken Kesey); explore spirituality (thank you, Ram Dass and Stephen Gaskin); go back to the land (thank you, *Mother Earth News*); and design a new future (thank you, *Whole Earth Catalog*).

The back-to-the-land season was in the early 1970s, right on schedule for alternative boomers. A group of friends and I lived for three years on fourteen acres in Rhinelander, Wisconsin, which is up there with Barrow, Alaska, in subzero temperatures. I went because I wanted to learn what an Ivy League education failed to teach me—how to walk on this earth like I belonged here, foraging, hunting, raising, and butchering animals and other fundamental arts of living. One of the group had bought the land sight unseen. We arrived with high ideals and a thorough lack of knowledge, only to discover that our homestead was a logged-out cranberry bog with just one acre above the water table.

We built a Depression-era Civilian Conservation Corps–style corduroy (log and sand) road from the blacktop to our island of high ground, and stuck a sign at the entrance: EGRESS. P. T. Barnum, father of the modern traveling circus, is famous for saying "There's a sucker born every minute." He suckered paying customers into moving through the sideshows as fast as possible by pointing them to one exotic feature after another. "This way to the tigress!" Oooooh. "This way to the Negress!" Aaaaah. Thus hooked, people would eagerly stream through the tent flap labeled THIS WAY TO THE EGRESS—which means "exit"—and find themselves out in the dust again. Our land was our egress from the conventional world and into our laboratory for a new society.

Everything was novel and exciting. I had a learning field day—quite literally because we needed to carve a field out of the forest to grow a garden. We cleared a half acre of scrawny alders and lodgepole pines with a bow saw and a machete. It was barely above the water table, so we dug drainage channels with a posthole digger. Even so, what we had looked nothing like "soil." It looked like a devastated clear-cut. We needed something akin to a plow.

Rhinelander is known for the Hodag, a mythical doglike snorting creature seen only by drunk hunters in the woods. To find our "something like a plow," we went first to the dump (an open, shopable pit down the road), then to the *Hodag Shopper*, the local trading rag. There we found a "perfectly good, just needs a little TLC" rototiller that Joe Dominguez, one of the community members, tinkered back to life. He rolled it out to the garden like a proud mama displaying her first baby in a pram. Instead of walking behind it, he stood on the back like a Roman charioteer, sinking the tiller's tines deep into the lumps and clumps as he rode triumphantly round and round the garden—spewing soil out the rear.

That our garden flourished was a miracle. Perhaps it was beginners' luck. Maybe it was the fact that we walked the garden daily—agricultural extension agent monographs in our dirty hands—like doctors on rounds, analyzing with our big brains what was happening to our peas and carrots.

I also traipsed through the woods with a copy of *Stalking the Wild Asparagus* by Euell Gibbons. I brought home fern fiddleheads and cattails to sample for dinner. Nothing tasted like chicken. It tasted like compost itself, and I was darn glad this was a three-year *voluntary* experiment in simple living.

We found a renegade piglet in the woods, named her Piggy Sue, fed her table scraps, and scratched her ears all summer. In early winter our neighbor Farmer Gray—a furniture salesperson turned farmer—helped us shoot and butcher Piggy Sue.

Farmer Gray became our mentor and benefactor in many ways. He'd hoped his children would stay on the eighty acres he'd bought with his savings to live his own "back to the land" dream of a self-sufficient farm. Instead they'd all skedaddled to Wausau and Madison as soon as they could, and our group of passionate young oddballs became "heirs" to his knowledge about hunting, butchering, canning, freezing, growing, harvesting, and more. After Sue he helped us butcher Dr. Buck, the deer that had been eating our garden; Jane Doe, the doe a hunter shot illegally and left for the coyotes; as well as a raccoon and rabbits. We cut Sue, Jane, and Dr. Buck into chops and roasts and stored the wrapped pieces in Farmer Gray's freezer over the winter—getting a package every Sunday for dinner. The rest of the week the meat would become soups and stews and toppings for beans and rice or part of meat sauces for pasta.

Farmer Gray's wife, Pat, helped us learn to cook what we'd killed. The secrets to making all types of game edible were (1) to cut out the scent glands that snaked between the hide and flesh, and (2) mountains of chopped tomatoes and garlic.

Farther down the road were Marty and Beulah, an old Lithuanian couple who took pity on us but also liked us. On our first visit they brought a dusty bottle up from the cellar, uncorked it, poured it, and told us to try it. It tasted like fine sherry. Dandelions, they proclaimed, pleased as punch to stump us. Back down they went for another bottle, this time a deep red, uncorked it, poured it, and watched us—now quite drunk—make appreciative smacking sounds with our lips.

Beets, they said, waggling their heads with pride. And so it was that I learned to make wine, which I did by the garbage-pail-ful in the woods. Beulah also taught me how to can food, which seemed like sex—wondrous and dangerous. Something could explode. Go awry. Start new life growing in your body, namely, botulism.

We would have harvested wild rice, which grew in the lakes all around, if it hadn't been the exclusive privilege of the Menominee Indians. We did buy it, though, along with fifty-pound sacks of potatoes, which, if I remember right, cost about five dollars each. We also always had a fifty-pound bag of field beans on hand, which may well have been grown in Wisconsin.

We ate plenty of that era's anywhere food too. Sacks of brown rice. Cans of tuna at three for a dollar (and still six ounces). Ketchup, though, we eventually learned to make from our own abundant tomatoes. Spaghetti. Blocks of yellow cheese. Flour for baking bread and making pancakes.

That Rhinelander experiment wasn't about 10-mile eating. It wasn't about "local" or "organic" as philosophies of life. It just happened to include lots of local food because we were bent on growing our own. We composted by feeding Piggy Sue. We enriched our soil via a load of pig manure delivered via belching tractor and jerry-rigged trailer from a half-blind pig farmer down the way, a recluse in Coke bottle glasses who spoke, if at all, in three-word sentences. The result may have been local, but the intent was survival.

Would my current experiment be much different?

Yes! In three ways:

First, this was a partnership between an eater and a feeder. I wasn't a spring chicken anymore, and had no desire to prove my prowess as a producer. Growing all my own food was not the great adventure I wanted in my sixties. As it turned out, this eater-feeder partnership led to one of my most profound transformations. Had I grown my own I would have missed it.

Second, I wasn't "leaving civilization." I would be eating Tricia's food in the context of what I call my plain vanilla people box—a split-level classic—in a subdivision in a village that's a twenty-minute ferry ride from Everett, Washington, home to three nuclear-powered aircraft carriers at the Naval Station Everett. As it turned out, this was crucial to the value of the experiment, as I was showing how you can "drop in" to eating local food rather than "dropping out" to the land.

Third, and this was a doozy, the world had changed in ways that make local food a crucial new normal rather than a quaint back-to-the-land season of a young person's life.

Back to the Land Versus Earth Day

As I was dropping out, going back to the land and within to find myself, others of my generation were dropping in to politics. While I was breaking apart assumptions and surmounting the significant challenges of living in a community and on the land, others were busting up different concrete—taking on the complacency of our upbringing and the dawning awareness that our new consumerist way of life had dark shadows: oil spills, poor air quality, pollution, and "the silent spring" of declining biodiversity thanks to pesticides, among other toxicities and injustices.

My generation's signature was a belief that we could change the world. Some of us, like me, went to the woods to live—as Thoreau exhorted—intentionally, so that when we died we would not discover we had not lived. Others went to the teach-ins on Earth Day, exhorted by Gaylord Nelson and Denis Hayes to protest the enemies of nature and protect mother earth. Back then there was still a choice between fight or flight. There was an "away." The population was only three and a half billion. Now it has doubled. Back then humanity was living well within the ecological means of the earth. Now our ecological footprint has increased by 250 percent. We are deep in ecological debt, yet, like so many debtors, we can't seem to slow down. Now we are consuming 1.4 planets' worth of resources every year. Our carbon footprint has also doubled.

The amount of land paved over to build houses, cities, and roads has increased by 75 percent; 75 percent more forests are felled now for paper and wood; 85 percent of our fisheries have collapsed. Carbon in the atmosphere has gone from 320 parts per million to nearly 400 ppm (350 ppm, according to climate scientist James Hanson, is the upper limit to keep a stable climate).

That first Earth Day and subsequent ones passed me by as I was living story number one—retreat and create—in the woods and later in the desert in southern Arizona, without phone, running water, a well, or an appetite for politics.

In 1980 I began to reengage. In a small way, my friends and I had been on a hero's journey—a quest to find the true gold of life beyond the safe and comfortable. Through our experiences we believed we had found something true, real, and of proven value to others: our approach to money and stuff that offered freedom through practical skills, frugality, and guts and through a larger purpose, service, and creativity. We taught the first "transforming your relationship with money" seminar in our living room, then in church basements and community centers, and eventually in auditoriums holding four hundred people. In short order, the demand outpaced our abilities. Overwhelmed, we re-created the seminar as an audio and workbook course, and let it travel around the world while we stayed home.

After all those years out of the mainstream, emerging again to teach was quite heady. But my heart wasn't on fire until the end of the decade. It didn't seem enough to simply help people one at a time. I had a thirst to understand how our personal strategy for change dovetailed with the big changes afoot in the world. Then I attended the Globescope Pacific Assembly in 1989. This first U.S. conference on a new idea—sustainable development—seemed just the place for a crash course in global issues. As I listened to the lectures and workshops, a tsunami of terrifying data swept over me about the state of the world.

It was like I was handed a big, blazing "While You Were Out" slip on which were written three bullet points:

- exponential growth
- overshoot and collapse
- limits to growth

These three horsemen of the environmental—civilizational, even—apocalypse are now referred to as the "triple crisis." For me it was a triple whammy.

It's in my nature to take ideas seriously, and these three big ones went right into my gut as shock, then into my heart as overwhelm, and then into my do-it-yourself head as a passion to act. If these terms are not familiar to you, read the next three sections. If they are, you can skip them.

Exponential Growth

A benign and beneficial name for exponential growth is "the magic of compound interest." You've seen the curves—maybe in a high school class, maybe in college, maybe in a sit-down with your financial planner. Let's say your wealthy aunt gives you $10,000 as a high school graduation present and you put it in the bank at 5 percent interest. In ten years with straight 5 percent interest you'd have $10,500. But if the interest was compounded (each month you get 5 percent on a new amount—capital plus accumulated interest), you'd have $16,500. By year 14 you would have doubled your money; the rule of thumb is that 7 percent interest doubles your base amount in ten years. In year 50 you'd have $122,000. Wait one more year and you'd earn another $5,400 in interest. This accelerating annual return is called "exponential growth."

Imagine a pond with one lotus atop a lily pad. Imagine that the lilies double daily. Day 2 there are two lily pads. Day 3 there are four. Day 4 there are eight. Say the pond will fill with lotuses atop lily pads by day 30. It's not until day 27 that the pond is just one-eighth full, a lovely lotus patch at the edge. Day 28 the pond is 25 percent covered. Next day it's 50 percent covered. Only half? Day 30 it's full. Growth creeps until it goes exponential. By the time we wake up, it's too late.

Exponential growth is great for your money. Not so great for finite systems. Like the earth.

We've seen these exponential growth curves for CO_2 in the atmosphere. And for population. Benign in the beginning. Devastating left unattended. Even though I had lived as low impact a life as you can imagine, just by inaction I had been complicit with these rising curves. I could see that by minding my own business I'd let these curves climb from yellow to orange to red alert through mere inattention. This dropped me back into the real world with a resounding thud.

Overshoot and Collapse

Day 30 the pond hits lily-carrying capacity, the term for the natural-resource limit for any species.

Day 31 the pond goes from lily-carrying capacity to lily overshoot. From growing freely, they hit a wall, crowd one another out, and collapse the system on which they depend.

Ecologists use this term—overshoot and collapse—to describe a condition in natural systems when one species, for whatever reason, takes advantage of an abundant food source, multiplies, eats through the supply, and then dies off.

You could say terminal cancer is a good example of exponential growth, overshoot, and collapse. Rogue cells grow and die in our bodies all the time, but for some reason—stress, diet, heredity, habits, toxins, bad luck—our resistance might be weakened, allowing that little cancer posse to grow. From the cancer's point of view, the body itself is a fantastic food source. Unchecked, the happily multiplying cells eventually take over a vital organ, causing the whole system to collapse, killing the cancer along with the body.

Overshoot and collapse is also the classic boom-and-bust business cycle, like the tech bubble or the housing bubble, where prices skyrocket beyond the underlying value of the commodity until the house of cards tumbles. Bankruptcy is another example, where the level of debt outstrips the ability to earn enough to pay the bills. You overshoot your personal financial means. Collapse is the outcome of overshoot.

Humanity sent the earth into ecological overshoot in 1986, according to the estimates of the Ecological Footprint, a very complex calculation of resource use based on the very simple idea that our consumption—from food to energy to furniture to housing—uses a measurable amount of "planet": water, land, animals, vegetables, minerals, materials. Your sofa, for example, has wood, cotton, perhaps brass tacks. All those can be weighed to determine the bit of the planet that is now embodied in this piece of furniture. Everything in your house can similarly be weighed. And in your driveway. And on your street. Everything counts—and can be counted by weight.

Since 1986 we have been using more planet each year than can be regenerated. We are overdrawing our ecological bank account, and going ever deeper into eco-debt. We have only one planet, so eventually this debt will crash systems. Which, as we've seen, is exactly what is slowly happening.

Limits to Growth

A team of brilliant young systems experts at MIT first sighted the shoals of human overshoot fifteen years earlier, in 1974. Their telescope, as crude as Galileo's, was a computer simulation of resource flows. Their data suggested that right about now our environmental ship would start scraping the bottom, and by midcentury our great growth economy enterprise would scrape the ground. The prestigious Club of Rome published their results as a book, *The Limits to Growth*. But no one believed their data. When we went into overshoot, few believed it. As George Bernard Shaw said, "It is the mark of a truly intelligent person to be moved by statistics." Clearly none of us has been very smart—we believe our senses, not predictions of what will happen decades hence.

Many great minds have offered explanations for why, in the face of the data, we have failed to act, but the fact is, we have lived out what Lao-Tzu observed centuries ago: "If you do not change direction, you may end up where you are heading."

To learn, in one weekend, about the titanic forces of exponential growth, overshoot and collapse, and the limits to growth was both terrifying and motivating. I saw the stark implications: our consumerist way of life was hitting the hard wall of planetary limits. In fact, we had already sailed off the cliff and were in free fall—we just thought we were flying. When I took my road less traveled I left the insanity behind, but these global problems affected everyone. There was no longer an egress—we were in this together.

True to boomer form, though, I also believed we could turn this tide, could lay new tracks to divert the runaway train. *We* can change the world if *we* can get *everyone* to do *the one thing* that would make all the difference. I believed this was the task of our generation, and failure was not an option. Drew Dellinger, in his poem "Hieroglyphic Stairway," asks:

It's 3:23 in the morning
and I'm awake
because my great great grandchildren
won't let me sleep
my great great grandchildren
ask me in dreams
what did you do while the planet was plundered?
what did you do when the earth was unraveling?

Because I had learned how to live frugally and joyfully on far less money than most thought possible—and because for ten years we had given seminars on our approach to money to thousands of people who reported a similar felicitous result (spending far less—on average, 20 percent less—and liking their lives better), I determined we'd get "everyone" to adopt this program.

The book I wrote with Joe Dominguez, *Your Money or Your Life,* came right out of that shock and determination. It became a major best seller and catapulted me from obscurity into the limelight! I truly believed that by the turn of the millennium we would have turned the tide of overconsumption.

For a decade, my coauthor and sidekick, Joe Dominguez, our equally committed team of friends, and I gave it our all. Even after Joe's death in 1997, the team soldiered on.

But the millennium arrived and the tide had not turned. Savings were down, debt was up, overshoot marched on. The only tide that had turned was an inner one. No longer able to pretend that I or even my generation would "fix" overshoot, I swung into the waiting arms of despair. We'd failed and were careening toward the wall, the fixed limits of ecological capacity.

For three years I kept going, though, like a bear keeps running after being mortally wounded. I tried new approaches to large-scale change. Some friends and I started the Conversation Cafés in Seattle. They eventually spread around the world. I helped bring forth the Pachamama Awakening the Dreamer Symposium. I wrote a book—not yet published—on rethinking freedom in a world with limits.

Cancer's Gift: Stop, Look, Listen

I needed to stop and face the limits to what one little human can do. It took a diagnosis, in 2004, of stage 3 colon cancer to do it for me.

It reined me in, slowed me down, and placed my attention in the present moment. Once again, after a decade of traveling, speaking, organizing, and mobilizing, I turned inward.

I actually did not have a will to live. I had a will to be alive, to experience my life again rather than fight to save it—or the world. I left all my positions of leadership. I left a comfortable home and friends who'd cared for me and moved into a small cabin above the beach to tend my soul—alone. I called it a cyber-shack: one room on dubious pilings, with a bed, bathroom, and kitchenette, and an Internet connection for my one thin thread of connection to others. There were rickety stairs to the beach, but I was so weak I could climb them only in stages. I ventured out for treatment and then dropped even that to simply be.

I was able to engage in a minute examination of the fear and frantic efforts that had driven me off my personal overshoot cliff. It's not that I had misread the data about the global problems. Or that my strategies for change were misguided. There was, however, something debilitating about how I dived into problems as if the only way to learn to swim were by almost drowning. I had been this way for as long as I could remember.

Never Leaving Well Enough Alone

One of my earliest memories, in fact, is precisely an example of this: to make up alternative games for me and my pals to play. At the age of five, I organized a school for some neighborhood kids in my bedroom, with me as the teacher. I believe this was before I could read, but I wanted to experience "school" before I was officially able to go.

Later I organized still more kids into a theater troupe and produced several open-air shows with that captive audience called parents. At summer camp I was also a theatrical producer, as well as the sponsor of costume parades. Once I could read and write, I started a family newspaper. At thirteen I did the same for my junior high, patiently typing each issue on mimeograph paper.

In college, my itch for "something else, I know not what" latched onto a year of study abroad. I made it happen—got professors to sign off on all the courses—even though Brown had no such program.

Fast forward and I'm on the road. Then living in extreme circumstances learning to survive on the land in an intentional community. Then writing an international best seller and promoting "enoughness" around the world. Then starting the Conversation Cafés. The Center for a New American Dream. Sustainable Seattle.

I don't take no for an answer when that bugle of purpose calls. At least I didn't until cancer pulled the rug out from under it all, and I sat for half a year facing the fears that drove me.

In that quiet I learned to let go rather than just get going to change the world. In this emptying I began to fill myself with a modest but authentic sense that even though the gathering eco-storm had not abated, my job was simpler than righting the whole ship of state. I found my intuitive heart and intuitive feet, an assurance that love is sufficient and I need to go only where I am led and love who is right there in front of me—without having any idea why. The cancer abated, my energy returned, and I once more went to a conference on the "big picture," where another "While You Were Out" slip got delivered. Peak Oil.

Peak Oil

"Peak Oil" is engineering-speak for the rising certainty that we have now burned half the available reserves of oil on the planet. The next quarter—like the Canadian tar sands—will be more difficult, risky, and expensive to extract. The last quarter we may never get to, as burning the prior quarter will surely send us into irreversible climate destabilization. Imagine our economy is a car. Even though we can still gas it up, running it drives us further toward environmental disaster. But not running it isn't an option either—our livelihoods depend on the engine's continuing to turn. To put it simply: if we step on the gas, we run out of planet. If we step on the brakes, people lose their jobs. Now what?

You will recognize this dynamic by now. Overshoot and collapse. This time for the very lifeblood of our industrial system. Oil. Stalled.

The global predicament was once more right in my face. Like a racehorse at the gate, like a bloodhound who catches a scent, everything in me wanted to race into the fray, inform and arm myself, and not take this news lying down. Yet I now knew that I had limits and that "all the king's horses and all the king's men" were not going to change what was already done. We were in the era of consequences, of adaptation. I did not know what to do. I could refrain from frantics (frightened antics) but I could not settle within. Surely something with integrity and wisdom could be done beyond mere acceptance.

Relocalization—preparing communities to thrive during the long transition from oil dependency to diverse, regional food, energy, and business systems—was the only big idea that made a little sense. But how? How to remake a ferry-dependent way of life designed around cheap oil and endless growth for its lifeblood? I could not imagine all our ferry commuters going to jobs at Boeing—one per car—squeezing back into a more rural way of life.

Partners in Caring

In 2007, I met a young couple, Britt and Eric, who also understood the gravity of the situation, the need for relocalization. They wanted to start a center where people could learn those necessary rural skills of growing food, cooking with the sun, building with mud, pacing life by the seasons. Just my kind of people, and right in time to partner on forming Transition Whidbey. In the box, you'll learn more about this approach.

Eric had inhaled with every baby breath his father's fierce desire for self-sufficiency and survivalist skills, so his young dreams were of being able to survive in the woods with nothing more than a knife. The hunter-gatherer lifestyle seemed the most natural way to live, and Eric eyed his uncle's sixty acres as a near perfect territory for a young buck to roam free. This shifted in college, though. Given that there are 7 billion people on the planet, sustainable settlements, not hunter-gatherer tribes, are the best way to collectively survive. Now his passion is for growing edibles, and he dreams of growing some portion of the many thousands of indigenous varieties. Give him a growing season and some ground and he'll be testing out crops and methods.

Britt, a wanderer and explorer, like me, has always had multiple interests, from shamanism to surfing. She met Eric in a class at Western Washington University in Bellingham—Eric was the student facilitator and Britt was the student—and felt a sense of destiny and deep love. Their vision of a sustainability center on Whidbey matched mine—and it was a concrete step we could take immediately.

I put my restless, creative mind on finding land to fulfill their vision—and include me in it. It was then that Ms. Frugality started saying wildly imprudent things, like "What's money for anyway?" and "I want to die with a dime in my pocket and not a day later" and (even worse) "I can take out a home equity loan. Why not?" Clearly I was in love with the vision and these passionate young people.

We almost bought a ten-acre property with another couple, but the deal fell through. I then tried to buy a hundred-year-old church with a parsonage, three acres, a big open sanctuary perfect for Conversation Cafés, classes, film nights, and social events, and a downstairs kitchen where we'd make soups and can vegetables in the fall. Again the deal fell through. My angels were hard at work! But the question remained: if my young friends and I couldn't relocalize, how could a whole island?

Transitioning Us All

Thankfully for my future financial security, I finally found a community-organizing strategy that wouldn't drain my life's savings. It was the Transition Town approach to relocalization.

Britt, a dozen others, and I helped start a Transition initiative on our island, with my silently swearing that I would keep myself in check and not drive myself off the cliff.

Aaah. I was now swimming in a current that made sense, that merited my energy. Started by the understated but ever-optimistic permaculture educator Rob Hopkins, the simple approach to intentionally powering down communities spread first in the UK and by now around the world. It's a head, heart, and hands approach.

Head is understanding—and helping neighbors understand—the climate, resource, financial, and energy challenges bearing down upon us.

Heart is unleashing the now-pent-up passion of communities to "Do something!"—to discover and get going on a less consumptive, more abundant way of life, one that runs on local sun, local soil, local industry, local love.

Hands is doing it—growing food, growing local currencies, growing businesses, encouraging pedal power, educating the public, changing ordinances, and hosting potlucks and parties and parades.

Within mere months we'd attracted a hundred-plus people, ready to act—and then we muddled through trying to organize that energy into a single engine—not easy with my unherdable neighbors. For all the good we were doing, though, we seemed a day late and a dollar short. We'd barely scratched the surface.

Pam Mitchell's Food Calculations

I turned to Pam Mitchell, a market gardener, to help me gauge our capacity here on Whidbey Island to feed ourselves. Her back-of-the-envelope calculations presented a pretty dire picture. Looking at her numbers I thought . . . We're toast.

Pam is a rare farmer. She didn't inherit land. She didn't buy land. She doesn't technically even rent land. She partnered with the owners, producing food for them in exchange for a (hefty) portion of the crop. I know this is called sharecropping in other parts, which is just this side of slavery. But Pam's strategy is canny to the max. She farms with no land debt, allowing herself to live on the proceeds of her farmers' market sales rather than plowing profits back into owning land.

Her arrangement is maintaining the events and flower gardens during the summer months and then cleaning up, moving plants if necessary, broadcast fertilizing, manuring, and replacing the irrigation system in the winter months, in trade for a residence in the barn, the processing room downstairs, and the quarter-acre vegetable garden / greenhouse space.

She has an engineer's mind, a love for vegetable production, and the good sense to seek out a "sharecropping" model that worked brilliantly, called SPIN-Gardening.

After years of tweaking the model, she has a precise system, a precise mix of growth medium for her seedlings, a precise selection of seeds, and a precise grow light system to produce vibrantly healthy starts for her gardens—and her customers. Her beds are built according to a successful formula as well. They are strung with watering tape, and soon after planting, uniformly gorgeous healthy vegetables march in straight lines, proud and ready to be harvested.

Having managed to support herself through gardening alone— after giving up her fall-back job at Boeing—Pam thought to train others in her methods. Enter Tricia, my soon-to-be feeder. She attended Pam's course on her high production and precision method and was well disposed when Pam and Laurie Carron (architect turned wannabe farmer) approached her with a proposal to start a CSA garden on the land she and her husband, Kent, had just bought. Tricia went one further. She wanted to be a partner in the business. In February 2008 they broke ground and started building beds with half a dozen volunteers. By June they had twenty-five customers.

Tricia was no stranger to growing food. She grew up in Ohio in one of those heartland families where the grandparents still had a large kitchen garden and canned in the fall to provision the family for the winter months.

Tricia and her husband-to-be, Kent Ratekin, met in 2004, got sparky, and were inspired to build a life together on their many walks in the woods. He too was from Midwest stock, and he was also a student of Rudolf Steiner, the father of biodynamic gardening (as well as of Waldorf education and many other spirit-infused arts). So it was natural for them to imagine buying a property and growing some food. They looked for just the right place and found a ten-acre parcel where a woman had raised seven children and countless chickens, dairy cows, and horses—all of which had amply fertilized sunny fields. The place was infused with love—and fertility. They made an offer, it was accepted, and they became not just occupants of the land but stewards.

Eventually Laurie went back to architecture and Tricia and Pam decided to each farm half the land independently and ended the partnership, but still, the spread of SPIN-Farming had started.

Pam went on to set up a garden on a different woman's land. It

was part of her vision: to multiply the model on successive properties, getting ever more garden partnerships going. Others are ex-
perimenting with this model as well. City Grown, for example, is
farming using people's Seattle yards. There's genius in seeing that
grassland yards can be farmland. And Pam is certainly a genius of
the practical.

The Straight Truth

So it was logical that I'd turn to Pam to assess our actual capacity for
food self-sufficiency on the island when the economic and energy
crises brewing like off-shore hurricanes eventually swept ashore—
which we both agreed they would do. That's when she did that back-
of-the-envelope calculation of Whidbey Island's ability to feed itself.
Agricultural land times estimated production per acre of veggies and
fruits that grow well here times total calories we could grow a year
divided by population . . . equals . . . practically no food beyond the
abundant summer season.

"We'd survive for August. Maybe."

That is a very big *Uh-oh*. How do you actually change a whole
food system so that it can nourish us—at least two months a year,
then three? How do we wean ourselves from utter dependence on
food that seems to come out of nowhere, produced by nobody we
know?

I moved to Whidbey because it was—and still is—a politically
and socially progressive community, especially the south end of the
island, where cultural creatives and millennials, artists and shop-
keepers, live alongside the Boeing commuters and socially conservative congregations with respectful diversity. In terms of the big waves
coming, though, we were as blind as picnickers on the beach who
fail to see the tsunami rolling in.

The magnitude of the problem was not lost on Pam. In fact, she
saw her work as part of bringing South Whidbey back to its commercial farming roots so it could land on its feet.

Life Goes On

I mulled, asked questions, hosted community conversations, tried (nicely—we are so nice in the Pacific Northwest) to alert people to the dangers of inaction—and at the same time lived my daily life. Britt and Eric bought three acres of open sunny land to farm. I partnered with another midlife woman to buy a house big enough for two solitary people—and then started a home-based teleclass business to supplement my retirement income. I spent a year updating *Your Money or Your Life*. When it came out in 2008, I came out further from my cancer cocoon. I wrote articles, several blogs, and a chapter in a book about how we are going to live in this era of collapse.

Bringing It All Back Home

In all this time the question never left me about how any locale might feed itself once the big wave of the triple crisis arrived at our shores. I tried to stay calm, to wait and watch and support existing food self-sufficiency enterprises. My instinct—like a greyhound's—was to chase solutions around the track. My body said, No more chasing rabbits. I watched us slip—politely—away from sufficient action. Like Cassandra, I hated the party-pooper role and tried to relax.

Then there was plain old laziness. I was passionate about relocalization but as disinclined as the next guy to change my own eating habits. I certainly didn't want anyone meddling with my choices, relishing my private life and my freedom to not be a paragon of lifestyle virtue. Yet I knew, deep down, that I was simply hiding, that my integrity would eventually out me. I was down to the only life I had any control over, the only human subject I could actually enroll in any experiment.

All this wore my will down to the point where I knew I didn't know, and I was willing to try one simple thing, not attempt everything. Stripped of all my big ideas, I was ready to do something real.

In hindsight, I see that my best work comes when I've exhausted my big ideas and I arrive at a small challenge to my personal integrity—to living the values I hold most deeply.

So there you have it. Tricia's trajectory and mine intersecting on the Fourth of July and striking this unusual deal that I would be her guinea pig in September.

I was ripe for such an experiment in radically living my values. Not changing the world but changing one little habit—where I source my food—for just thirty days.

As I went through the summer planning for my plunge into hyperlocal eating, I began to get glimmers of what would by the end of the experiment be vividly clear. Our global food system is very much like our global money and stuff system, only grittier, more real and fundamental to our survival. Growing populations with growing tastes for complex foods have sent us into food overshoot, leaving us with the food-poor, the food-rich, and a food-compromised earth. I began to wonder if it would be possible to transform our relationship with food the way Joe and I transformed our relationship with money. Can we live again within the means of the earth? What is the role of personal change in that task? Might our lives gain meaning and dignity by linking our personal change to the collective change of our times?

July 4, 2010, I was distinctly healthy and well established in my new life on my little island. My own crisis well past, I was ready to open the door again to this global crisis—and how I might help. Thanks to Tricia, it turns out that meant opening my mouth again. Not to speak, but to eat.

Now It's Your Turn: Your Food Future

Just like we all have food histories, we have food futures. What do you believe about the future? Do your assumptions about the future affect how you live today? Would you rather not think about the future because it's all too scary and uncertain? Do you love thinking about the future, planning and dreaming? Have you changed anything because of your assumptions?

In this chapter I've laid out my view of the future, which has motivated my work for change and my life work as a sustainability activist and educator. Here are some questions to help you unlock your thinking about the future. As with food messages, focusing on your beliefs, assumptions, and research data can help you shape a food future for yourself—and for our world.

- What helps you think about the future?
- What do you assume about the future?
- Do you believe your children will be as food abundant and secure as you are? More? Less? Why?
- Do you believe that the big global forces—peak oil, climate change, financial instability—will actually affect *your* food future?
- If yes, what steps are you taking now? Which ones do you mean to take but haven't gotten around to yet?
- People who relocalize do some of these things. What steps make sense to you, given your sense of the future?
  — rethink where you live
  — rethink how you earn and spend money
  — grow or expand a garden
  — get a plot in a community garden
  — join a CSA (Community Supported Agriculture farm)
  — put some solar panels on your roof
  — change appliances
  — weatherize your home
  — join or start a local Transition group
  — influence politics
  — write and speak about the importance of relocalization
  — learn how to repair simple—or complex—things
  — form/join networks of mutual aid

Your Dream Food Future

Write anything, from one word to a page, about your vision of a desirable food future, one you want for yourself, your children, and your grandchildren—a foundation for generations to come. What can you be doing today to make that future a reality? What can you dedicate yourself to, in your daily habits and in your community and professional work? What new food rules can you set for yourself to help move this process along?

HOW TO START A TRANSITION TOWN GROUP

Personal change is challenging enough, but to change your community you need to work in groups. Transition Towns was the approach I found. Here's a very short course on how to start a Transition Town Group; if you are going to actually do it, you'll want to get The Transition Companion *by Rob Hopkins, the originator of the approach.*

Transition Towns is a citizen-led approach to bulking up community resilience, a tool for people who wake up to the power communities have to respond proactively as global resources, finance, and climate prove ever more unstable. It is both improvisational—arising from the creativity and guts of local people who care—and systematic—a recipe with ingredients that together generate ever more food, energy, and economic and cultural community resilience. It's both easy—just pick it up and get going—and difficult—odds of success improve with good leadership, good group-process skills, a volunteer or paid coordination team, good community-organizing mojo, and patience.

WHAT DO PEOPLE DO WHEN THEY "TRANSITION"?

They first get a group together to talk about the challenges of our times and how to get their community engaged. They talk to a lot of people about the issues and possibilities—from neighbors to government officials. They organize some community events to network existing groups and form new ones to get some projects going. Often it's a monthly potluck or a community garden or a rural-skills series or a seed bank or trade/barter systems. Above this low-hanging fruit are bigger challenges: community-asset mapping and developing a plan for the near future, when fossil fuel will be dear yet local communities will be thriving. A lot of this depends on people sticking with it, finding a way to be relevant to many sectors of the community, having on balance more fun than frustration, constant learning, and skill building. It is the work of a lifetime, really, because if we are lucky the transitions will happen not in a scary few years but in a graceful adaptive process.

THE 7 GUIDING PRINCIPLES OF TRANSITION TOWNS:

1. *Positive visioning*—Generate a compelling picture of where we are headed, not just a compelling analysis of what is going wrong.
2. *Awareness*—Give communities the best current information about the challenges posed by resource and economic crises, trusting them to see the implications and act appropriately.
3. *Openness and inclusion*—Make participation clear and available to all sectors of the community.
4. *Enable sharing and networking*—Through all the wonderful tools of social networking—online and off—allow the community to celebrate the successes, see the failures, and jump in where they feel called.
5. *Build resilience*—Engage in empowering and visible projects in every sector of community life.
6. *Inner and outer transition*—Outer change makes waves in our minds and heart. Sharing our journeys is part of the process.
7. *Subsidiarity*—A big word for making decisions as close to those affected as appropriate. Relocalization inherently means people-in-community power.

Try These Recipes

Lisa Morrill and Chef Vincent Nattress shared recipes for this chapter.

Lisa Morrill owns The Braeburn Restaurant in downtown Langley. Since we've just considered our ecological footprint, exponential growth, and overshoot, I thought we'd need some comfort food right about now.

Ma's Meatloaf

9 eggs

5 tablespoons heavy cream

½ cup Worcestershire sauce

2 cups organic ketchup

8 to 12 slices dried rustic bread, torn into small pieces

2 cups sun-dried tomatoes, julienne cut

1 large yellow onion, roughly chopped

5 tablespoons fresh Italian parsley, chopped

3 tablespoons fresh oregano, chopped

3 tablespoons fresh rosemary, stemmed and chopped

10 tablespoons crushed garlic

2 pinches salt

3 pinches black pepper

5 pounds 3 Sisters grass-fed ground beef

Preheat the oven to 350°F.

Combine the eggs, heavy cream, Worcestershire sauce, ketchup, and bread, stir, and let sit about 3 minutes.

Add the sun-dried tomatoes, onion, fresh herbs, garlic, and salt and pepper, mix, then add the ground beef and mix well.

Scrape the mixture into two well-oiled 9 x 5-inch loaf pans.

Bake for 1½ hours. Remove and let cool.

Lisa says:

At The Braeburn, we specialize in great Pacific Northwest breakfasts and lunches made fresh with only the best ingredients. We use local and organic product whenever available and are fortunate to have a bounty of wonderful farms around us to utilize.

We make our meatloaf to serve as a sandwich, though it's also delicious as an entrée alongside herbed mashed potatoes and some local greens. Our sandwich is a ½-inch slice of meatloaf (grilled) on toasted Scala bread from the Essential Baking Company, with lettuce, tomato, alfalfa sprouts, and a light spread of mayo.

Originally from a rural farming community in Vermont, I grew up watching my mother and my grandmother cooking with fresh vegetables and herbs from their gardens, fruit from the patches in the backyard, milk and cheese from the dairy farm down the street, and fresh local meat from the animals raised in the pastures nearby. Living on Whidbey we are so fortunate to have similar farms and product available to us here. My vision when taking over The Braeburn was to utilize as much of that bounty as possible to make the food and menu items here feel like they came out of the kitchens I grew up eating in. Fresh, simple, and homemade with love.

Lisa's co-chef is Patrick Boin, whose chicken recipe you'll find in chapter 6. About him Lisa says, "I can't tell you how lucky I was to have Patrick walk through my door last year. He has been able to help make my 'vision' an actual reality here!" When you read his recipe, you'll know why she says this.

Now for an elegant recipe—using mostly local ingredients—from Chef Vincent Nattress, who grew up in Coupeville on Whidbey Island. He worked as a chef and culinary consultant around the world and then returned to Whidbey to live a balanced life with his wife and two daughters. In 2010 he founded the Whidbey Island Slow Food Convivium, which produces an exquisite local feast each year: the Taste of Whidbey. Combining his love of food and of farming, he and his wife bought a centrally located piece of land where they can grow fruits, vegetables, and poultry while she does yoga and he continues as a sought-after fine chef. I picked his salad recipe because Vincent's passion for Slow Food arises not just from his love for cooking but from his understanding of the links between industrial agriculture, climate change, and peak oil.

Salad of Fall Greens, Poached Hen's Egg, Walnut Vinaigrette

This warm salad is a great way to showcase our range-fed chicken eggs. The thing that is amazing about them, because our chickens are on grass every day of the year, is the color and richness of the yolk. While you could do a salad like this any time of the year, it is particularly good with heartier fall and winter greens, like those in the chicory family: endive, radicchio, escarole to name just a few. These slightly bitter greens make a flavor explosion when combined with the acidity of the vinaigrette, the sweetness of the walnuts, and the richness of the egg, which serves to richen the dressing as it incorporates. Two things to note: First, always buy the best red wine (or any flavor) vinegar you can get your hands on; good vinegar is not expensive and goes a long way, and the good stuff is so much more impactful than lesser-quality vinegar. Second, good walnut oil is expensive and all nut oils tend to go rancid quickly; store it in the refrigerator and always taste before using to make sure it is sound.

MAKES 4 SALADS

1 head escarole

2 Belgian endives

1 head radicchio

1 bunch watercress

1 large shallot, chopped

1 small garlic clove, smashed

2 tablespoons good-quality red wine vinegar

2 teaspoons honey

1 teaspoon Dijon mustard

salt and pepper

¼ cup pure olive oil

¼ cup walnut oil

1 tablespoon white vinegar (distilled or white wine)

4 hen's eggs

1 teaspoon finishing salt (like Maldon, Murray River, French *gros sel,* or
  fleur de sel)
1 cup walnut halves, toasted

Cut the escarole, endive, and radicchio into bite-sized pieces and soak them in cold water for 1 hour. This will crisp them up and go a long way to reducing any excess bitterness. Once they have soaked, drain them and spin them dry with a salad spinner. Trim, wash, and spin the watercress as well. All the greens should then be stored well covered with a damp towel in the coldest part of your refrigerator. They will hold well without noticeable browning if stored this way for up to a day.

For the vinaigrette, combine the shallot, garlic, red wine vinegar, honey, mustard, and salt and pepper to taste in a bowl. Place a damp towel, formed into an O, under the bowl, so that as you whisk the contents the bowl stays put. Whisk the ingredients well to combine, then allow it to sit and pickle for 2 to 5 minutes. Slowly add the oils, whisking continuously, to form a loosely emulsified vinaigrette. Taste the dressing and adjust the seasonings with salt and pepper. As no two oils and no two vinegars are the same, you may have to add slightly more vinegar or slightly more oil. The vinaigrette should be quite bright and acidic, but not overly so.

When you are ready to serve, bring 4 cups of water to a simmer in a small sauce pan. Add the white vinegar. Break the eggs into a small cup or ramekin and check to make sure there are no shell fragments in them. Stir the simmering water in a circular fashion, so it is moving gently. Carefully add the eggs to the simmering water and set a 4-minute timer.

Meanwhile, place the greens in a large bowl and dress with the vinaigrette, salt, and freshly cracked pepper. Hold back some of the vinaigrette to garnish the salads. Divide the greens between four plates, making a place in the center of each plate for the egg to land when it is done. Once the timer for the eggs goes off, check to see that they are poached to your liking—I like them quite soft; you will have your preference, but you certainly do not want the yolk fully cooked, as it is going to help make the dressing—then remove them with a slotted spoon and dab them dry with a clean towel. Place an egg on each salad.

Garnish each egg with the finishing salt and freshly cracked pepper. Sprinkle the walnuts around the salads. Drizzle the remaining vinaigrette over each egg and around the outside of each plate.

CHAPTER THREE

Yes! But How?

A Change of Date

Tricia and I first presumed we'd start the experiment in August—just four weeks away. On second thought—and there were a series of second thoughts—September looked better.

First, August meant I might not get to eat at Britt and Eric's wedding. Even though they'd committed to grow all the food and flowers for their wedding—and it had taken them two years to make good on that—my original bargain was to eat only what Tricia could grow. This was one wedding where I did not want to miss the food.

Second, Tricia and I were both, frankly, worried about whether I'd have enough to eat and wanted more time to adjust to what we'd set in motion. While I could not have found a better person to provide the bulk of my food than Tricia, when I contemplated a month with no meat, I knew that would tip the adventure too far into the austerity zone. Even with the eggs she promised, even with plenty of hearty root crops like beets and turnips, carrots and potatoes, I still could not imagine a month almost completely without protein from meat, beans, nuts, grains, or dairy. The idea of thirty days of eating only vegetables, reminiscent of the Irish potato famine, got me thinking. Hard.

Which is how I came up with adapting the challenge from an exclusively Tricia diet to a 10-mile diet. As Tricia and I live six miles from each other (shorter as the crow flies), and the number ten felt nice and round, I suggested we include in our experiment any food grown within ten miles of my home. We'd stick to her food as much as humanly (and humanely) possible, but I was free to seek out meat and dairy within that narrow radius. At that moment I had no idea how far ten miles would get me, but I was sure I could find some locally raised and butchered meat. As I said, there was a sheep pasture by my house, and cattle grazed in a field just up the hill; each spring calves and lambs gamboled around, grew fat on lush grass, and disappeared . . . presumably not just to the toasty barn for the winter. Surely some of that meat would be available.

Provisioning for the 10-mile month took the entire month of August. Let's do before-and-after snapshots of how I ate.

Exhibit A: The Everywhere, Every-Reason-in-the-Book Eater

Before my 10-mile diet experiment, I was your typical food slut. While I had your standard good dietary intentions, I "ate around," so to speak. I put all sorts of dubious things in my mouth—like day-old anything and fried mystery meat from street vendors.

I had (and still have) an inconsistent range of values governing where I shopped, what I bought, what I ate for meals, and what I ate voraciously at odd hours with a glazed look in my eyes. Here are my criteria for what I ate (you'll notice they don't make a matched set):

• *Cheese.* Anything with cheese. Crackers, vegetables, nachos, toast, salad.

• *Simplicity.* Simple to cook. Simple to eat. No multistage recipes. No recipes that take you to the store at five P.M. for a magic ingredient. No multicourse meals. No complex sauces that have a possibility of curdling or running. Simplicity could mean a garden salad or an apple or oatmeal. It could also mean eating ice cream from the carton in a dark kitchen lit only by the light from the freezer.

• *Frugality.* How am I frugal? Let me not obsessively count the ways. Frugality isn't just a set of techniques for me. It has been a lifelong sport, art, science, talent, challenge, strategy, and necessity. It was also part of my *Your Money or Your Life* persona for two decades; it wasn't a jacket I could take off. It was a tattoo. As a shopping criteria it can lead me to eating some pretty lifeless food, but combined with simplicity it could mean buying in bulk, buying on sale, buying from the day-old-but-perfectly-good bin. It definitely means knowing what I like and stocking up when it goes on sale. It also means shopping, cooking, and eating such that I rarely throw food away.

• *Healthy.* Combine that with simple and you get fresh fruits and vegetables. Combine it with frugal and simple and you get the same foods—on sale. Combine it with dietary recommendations that almost every omnivore follows and you get wild salmon, free-range chicken, and dairy.

• *Ethics.* From time to time, some industrial practice or another has so dismayed me that I've simply stopped eating that food. When Donella Meadows (coauthor of *Limits to Growth*) explained her research about the impact of shrimp harvesting on the mangroves in Thailand, I simply stopped eating shrimp. When I read John Robbins's first book, *Diet for a New America,* I stopped eating beef for ten years. I wasn't virtuous in general. I was aware through friends of the hidden costs of these foods—the devastation to ecosystems, the cruelty, the diseases managed by antibiotics, the conditions of the workers. Selective conscience.

• *Low-calorie.* Yes, this is a food group. Given my druthers I'd crunch on almonds rather than celery any day of the week, but I stock up on foods I can eat in volume without gaining bulk. You have to eat your celery before you can have your dessert.

• *Preference.* This is in a class all its own, and it can trump all of the above when I am in the presence of my favorite ice cream, salad dressing, crackers, nuts, cereal, bread, soft drink, chips, tea, coffee, and tropical fruit—you know, the basic food groups. If any are on sale, then I stock up and get a frugality point or two.

• *Convenience.* Road food. Airport food. Fast food. Sometimes a girl's just gotta eat what's easy.

• *Comfort.* Meatloaf. Greasy chicken from the deli. Rice or baked potato with butter. Cashews. Cocoa. Popcorn. When stressed or sad, these are my baby bottle.

- *Because it's there.* If I'm at a potluck or a party with hors d'oeuvres, I simply must try everything. And go back for seconds.

I actually felt good about how I ate. It was healthy enough, cheap enough, ethical enough, yummy enough, and free enough of obsession that I could enjoy myself and not overthink it.

Exhibit B: The Everywhere Shopper

As a frugality queen in the 1990s, I considered smart shopping my crowning glory. I gushed hundreds of times in the media about how I lived sumptuously on, at that time, well under one thousand dollars a month. "I buy my freedom with my frugality," I said over and over—and while it's true, it's also true that my frugality was a habit, an obsession sometimes, and even a profession. After all, I wrote a best seller on the topic!

Being frugal, I had no qualms about phoning around to comparison-shop, shopping at those reviled big box stores, reading sale ads, clipping coupons, stocking up on loss leaders, cruising the discounted food bins, and knowing by heart the normal prices of hundreds of items so I could spot bargains. My mind was a nonstop cash register—registering the cost of everything. I was a volume eater and a value shopper.

Even after moving out of the house in Seattle where I lived with my hyperfrugal New Road Map Foundation team, my habits persisted and I aimed to feed myself on less than two hundred dollars a month if I could—and I did.

The closest market to my home in Langley is the Star Store, a ten-minute walk from my door. Langley, ten minutes from the ferry but off the main road, is on the east side of the island, yet it faces north. A crook in the coast forms a harbor that drew the original inhabitants of the island to ship logs harvested from the interior off to Seattle to build the city. From those muddy streets and its logging-town roughness a century ago, Langley has evolved into "the village by the sea," attracting tourists to our galleries and shops on First Street, families to the safety for their kids, and retirees to our bluffs and hills with commanding water views. My house is on one of those hills in a subdivision where modest houses have surprisingly killer views.

Second Street is where we villagers do our daily rounds. The post office and library are at one end. I've been here long enough that if there's an item too big for my PO box, not all the clerks need my box number to fetch the package. The bank is at the other end of Second, and there too I don't need to pull out identification to cash a check. Across from the bank is our only general store—a cavernous thrift store linked to our food bank. Several restaurants and coffee shops flank the block between these upper and lower anchors, and if you sit in any of them long enough, a river of friends flows through for a cup of soulful conversation. And then there in the middle is the Star Store. Langley is such a small town that our market has a first and last name, and anyone who just calls it the grocery store is definitely not from these parts.

Fundamentally the Star Store is where we do our visiting and our business as well as our shopping. The triangle formed by the cheese, dairy, and meat displays is large enough for a good long conversation without completely blocking others. The little space by the two checkout lines is another meeting place, as is, of course, the produce section. Somehow the owners, Gene and Tamar, manage to be eclectic enough to please us all—snack addicts to health-food nuts. Having that price book still in my head, I can do a quick cruise of all the aisles, stocking up on bargains and a few must-have preferentials, like avocados. My menus track their sale ads, one week chicken and sliced cucumbers, another week fish and whatever fruit is a bargain.

The Star Store is where I most often shop and therefore most often ponder the "organic" question. Here's my inner calculus as I play Ms. Bobblehead in the produce section. To my left is organic. To my right is conventional. My rule of thumb has been that I buy organic if it is no more than 50 percent costlier than the regular version. Sometimes I push that closer to double the amount, but that mostly happens when I feel flush, virtuous, or am next to someone who tilts my conscience.

The Goose Community Grocery Store, a ten-minute drive door to door, is my other market, The Goose came out of a partnership between the sustainability-focused nonprofit Goosefoot and the grocer who runs the store. It's the rebirth of an old IGA market that had worn, dingy black-and-white linoleum tile floors, a small produce section, and a big dollar aisle. It suited the food-stamp volume-shopper crowd, but island activists asked for something closer to a food co-op with a bit of Whole Foods, Trader Joe's, and a fair trade coffee bar mixed in. Pleasing everyone was a tough job—especially if you include pleasing the bean counters (as in money, not beans). The market had to be financially viable or no one would get any of what they wanted.

How the Goose turned out reflects the needs of the old shoppers looking for value and volume, and the new shoppers looking for organic and bulk. It feels like Costco when you enter. To get to the produce, you have to walk the gauntlet of cartons stacked eight feet high with cutouts revealing the packaged foods on sale—the twelve-roll packs of toilet paper, the jugs of perfumed detergents, the boxes of sugary cereals, the cans of salty green beans and corn, the bags of wrapped candies.

You turn the corner, though, and you're in a fresh and bulk food section with more of a co-op feel. The vegetables are tended with care, always trimmed and beautiful. The bulk food manager will get you anything you want, in addition to stocking about five hundred items—literally from soup to nuts—including at least twenty kinds of grains and a dozen kinds of flour, a dozen granolas, a dozen types of dried fruits, and even tea and spices.

I used to do a lot of my shopping on The Dark Side, which is what we islanders call the mainland, a ferry ride away. My two big stops were Trader Joe's and Van's Produce.

Trader Joe's—or TJ's, to those who know him well—has my demographic nailed. The entryway is almost strewn with petals. Pots of orchids and big sprays of colorful bouquets greet the eye as you arrive. None of the floor-to-ceiling cartons of Costco—or the Goose. Free taste treats in the far corner of the store lead you by your nose (and mouth) through the aisles stacked high with artisan breads and packaged nuts, and frozen Yuppie food and vitamins and chocolate and cheeses—most of it easier on the wallet than any other grocery store. By the taste kiosk is an endless supply of coffee, free in two-sip cups. That'll get your shopper mind revving. Most of what I tended to buy there were preferentials, not essentials—but sometimes Mediterranean hummus feels like a necessity. The clerks probably all take comedy tests as part of the application process because they are charming. Sure, TJ's business model squeezes their suppliers until only one penny of profit is left in the grower's pockets, but I just couldn't get that injustice to stick in my mind once I walked through the portals and felt the pull of flavors plus frugality.

My other stop was usually Van's Produce in Seattle's International District. It's where the Chinese restaurateurs shop, and the other customers are mostly Asian. They have huge bags of dried shiitake mushrooms, strange long, hairy roots, and never-before-seen fruits, plus the standard vegetables you'd find in Chinese meals. Most items are 25 to 50 percent less than I'd pay on Whidbey—from farmers or grocers. The veggies often seem like seconds—imaginative shapes, hangdog limp, maybe bruised. They say it all comes from Mexico, which before the 10-mile diet didn't strike me as a problem. I usually left with twenty-five dollars' worth of produce, which would last me a week or more.

Here's another reason why Van's worked for me: volume. Like many compensatory eaters—we who eat to satisfy hungers that have nothing to do with the stomach—I sometimes crave a Niagara Falls flow of food down my gullet. Like most dieters, though, I need low-calorie volume or my personal volume will increase exponentially. And my frugality dictates that I do all this within my money as well as calorie budget. You can see why I always stopped at Van's when on The Dark Side.

I occasionally shopped the farmers' markets in the summer, but, to be honest, I went more for the socializing and music than the produce, jams, or soaps. I was what I call a three-beeter. That's a person who buys three beets at a farmers' market to get their local-food Girl Scout badge, but gets 99 percent of the rest of their calories from who-knows-where.

The problem for me with the farmers' market, as I said, was my hyperfrugality. Many of my eventual breakthroughs from the 10-mile diet came from crossing that long frugal-to-local divide. I now understand the forces that make the local cheese, meat, and veggies more expensive and am more committed to the well-being of my farmers than to scrimping. In fact, I learned many ways to think about the cost of beets that makes the farmers' market beets a flat-out bargain.

By the way, nothing on my shelves was going to be "in bounds" come September 1. All my frugal shopping, all my careful metering of chocolate and nuts and celery and popcorn, was about to stop. It was all . . . what do you call the opposite of local food? Food of unknown origin? Industrial food? Commercial food? Global food? Supermarket food? Approved by the FDA, so surely it's fit for human consumption food? Plastic food? Grown with slave labor, laden with chemicals, subsidized by man-eating lobbyist sharks food? Really, this kind of food is so normal it no longer needs a name. What a difference one hundred years makes. Back then, local was the norm, and what we take for granted today was fancy food, foreign food, rich people's food, and delicacies.

Even before I started my 10-mile diet, I was being forced to become even more conscious of food than if I were on a diet. Everything that seemed normal and insignificant rose up for reexamination.

I had not thought so comprehensively about diet since I'd been diagnosed with cancer.

Exhibit C: Diet and Cancer

When my tests came back positive for blood in my stool, the only dietary culprit I suspected was pumpkin seeds.

I was holed up in a cabin at the time, pecking away at a big book on "rethinking freedom in a world with limits." I wanted to challenge our current low-life sense of freedom as entitlement to do whatever we want, whenever we want without regard for the consequences. I wanted Americans to fall in love with limits, with everything that holds us together, that creates civility, that makes for fair play and justice and a healthy future. I sat day in and day out in the dripping Northwest woods writing, rewriting, and eating popcorn and pumpkin seeds to at least put my gnashing of teeth to good use. The words and metaphors lumbered across the pages like great dusty pachyderms. I just couldn't seem to present the idea of limits so that people would say "Mercy me, how could I have thought I wanted to have everything my way! I'd much rather share and share alike with the other six billion on this wee, precious planet."

The only distressing symptom I had was leg cramps in the early morning. I took potassium, magnesium, and calcium, but they persisted, stumping me enough to get me to the doctor, who gave me the stool test card, and told me to fill it out and come back. Result: blood in every sample. Suspecting that the volume of seeds and popcorn had somehow rubbed my colon raw, I ate white rice for a week and did the test again. Same results. Next came the colonoscopy. Then came the news no one ever wants to hear: you have cancer.

As it was colon cancer, you'd think I'd have made some link to diet, but I didn't. I told whomever came at me with their latest theory of food and cancer, "I eat kale on my hands and knees in the garden. I eat broccoli. If I had to limit myself to one food group, it would be 'green.'"

Still, I became a magnet for cancer-curing diet recommendations. Brown rice. Seaweed. Wheat grass juice. Juicing in general (one friend had a juicer delivered to my home as soon as she heard the diagnosis). Carrots, celery, greens, beets, cucumbers, ginger—send it all down the neck of the juicer and drink your way to health. Blueberries, bananas, cranberries. Orange food. Yellow food. Red food. Stop drinking coffee—but take it as an enema.

As I quietly assessed these diets for myself, I recognized in them the same mentality as in weight-loss diets: a pummeling of the flesh to fix a perceived problem.

Of course I preferred life to death and being fit over being fat. But the "fixing" mind leaves no room for the quieter, more difficult work of going within to find what's true. When you lose trust in yourself to know what is good for you and in your body as a self-healing, self-regulating miracle, you become the patsy for every quack cure and ersatz diet. So I thanked everyone for their concern and told them to keep their good ideas to themselves.

Traditional peoples, I also reasoned, didn't have to wonder about food choices. Some based their diets on corn, some on wheat, some on rice, some on whale blubber, and you know what? If any of those diets was wrong, none of us would be here today. Chew on that. One great wonder of the world is that our bodies can transform just about anything that isn't poison into food for us—day in and day out.

No, cancer didn't change anything about my diet.

Setting the Table for My 10-Mile Month

As the cancer crisis receded, the triple crisis heaved up on the horizon, groaning like a distressed frigate about to come apart at the seams. I couldn't ignore it.

Transition Whidbey had mobilized a lot of energy. Hundreds attended our monthly events called Potlucks with a Purpose—a magic combination of eating, socializing, networking, and an open mike where people offered their surplus, asked for what they needed, celebrated their wins, and announced their events. A lecture would fill the minds once the body and heart were satisfied—most often with information that would jolt us into awareness and action. At the end, new or ongoing action groups had time to meet.

Even so, these potlucks did not *fix* anything. My inner "Uh-oh, we're in deep doodoo" meter was still in the red; we weren't moving far enough or fast enough to make difference enough in time. To add insult to injury, I wasn't doing it either. No longer my old paragon of sustainability virtue, I had allowed a complex and costly life to grow up around me. In my old community house, shared with half a dozen people, I had only a few hundred square feet to call my own. Now I owned a two-thousand-square-foot split-level people box—and lived here alone! Back then, my ecological footprint was four acres, on par with a Mexican.

Now it was seventeen acres, which means if everyone lived as I do, it would take four planets to provide for us. I was far from integrity, given what I knew of overshoot. The pressure to either jettison my values or do something about them increased. Thanks to Tricia's challenge I was now accountable to someone else—and a *very* generous person at that. I would finally make a *very*-good-faith effort to eat *very* locally. The 10-mile diet did what cancer could not: get me to engage enthusiastically with limiting my last bastion of willful disregard for the consequences of my actions: food.

I was a bit nervous, very curious, and strangely relieved, like when you finally square your shoulders, march into your garage, and start cleaning out everything that's been long forgotten but not gone. The task has been waiting for you. The effort to ignore it has worn you down. It got so that when people admired your home, you thought, Ah, but you haven't seen the mess in my garage.

Now, to stock my fridge and freezer for September.

Satisfying My Meat Tooth

In late July, driving over to set up for Britt and Eric's wedding, I passed some green fields I'd always admired in an "Isn't my island just the prettiest place?" kind of way. A small hand-painted sandwich board by the driveway read, MEAT SALE TODAY 10–2. I was no longer a casual Sunday driver. I was driven—and I swerved in. It turned out to be the Long Family Farm.

The 200-acre farm has been in the family for five generations. It all started in 1912 with a Dutchman, Claus Brower, who came to those very fields in Maxwelton Valley where I was about to "score" some protein for September. Claus eventually married the widowed Nancy Long, who arrived from Montana with three sons in tow. The boys purchased 300 cull chickens from Percy Wilkenson's hatchery in Clinton and started their own farm next door. Over the years, the flock grew to 5,000 laying chickens and some cattle. After Claus's death, Joe Long grew the operation further to 130,000 chickens and more than 100 Angus cows. His son Leland and his grandsons, Robert and Loren, dropped the chickens, kept the cows. They now raise healthy 1,200-pound, two-year-old, grass-fed, and corn-grass-finished animals. A mobile slaughter truck humanely slaughters them, and then the carcasses go to be aged, cut, and wrapped by the nearest USDA-approved butcher (forty miles and a ferry ride away). Some is sold there and some is sold locally to restaurants, grocers, and individuals—like me that Saturday.

This five-generation history is part of the hope of our island. It reaches back to a time when we could actually feed ourselves with local foods—and did. Even New York City, if it went back five generations, would find similar hope—maybe not within ten miles, but certainly fifty. My own life began on that other island—Long Island—before Levittown transformed Nassau County's potato farms and pine forests into one of the first large-scale, low-cost subdivisions. I remember how they heralded Levittown as a miracle for the middle class, part of the optimism and rising affluence after World War II. No one at the time thought they'd miss those potato farms—and we haven't. Yet. But if feeding ourselves without access to cheap, easily produced oil means we all need to eat foods grown closer to home, it's good to know the lawns and parks and estates and hobby farms of Nassau County are still, in essence, soil that a new crop of young farmers—with support and education—could farm to help feed the city folk. The fact that farming close to where we live was once normal means it can be once again.

Go back further in time on Long Island and you'd meet tribes like the Canarsee, Rockaway, Merrick, and Manhasset. You'd see them gathering clams along the shore, fishing from their canoes and hunting in the forests for wild game. Much of their food was harvested without being cultivated, a rarity now, a reality for most of human history.

You'd see the same on our West Coast "long island"—Whidbey. The Duwamish, Snohomish, and Snoqualmie tribes flourished along this whole coastal region[1]—mostly summering here on Whidbey, following the seasonal foods—until the white settlers came 150 years ago, logging the island like a barber would give a buzz cut. With skirmishes and raids, the settlers gained ground until they drove the natives out. A road connecting south to north was built, then the bridge connecting Oak Harbor to the mainland, while ferries connected the south to Everett. A naval air station was built on some of the best farmland—because it was flat. Zoning and land-use policy, combined with the relatively cheap land on the island compared to the mainland, eventually dotted the countryside with five-acre hobby farms amid the remaining forests, small cities, and developments and a few large farms like Greenbank Farm and those on Ebey's Prairie, now preserved as a historical—and farming—reserve.

For most of human history, cities have been intimately involved in food production. Architect Carolyn Steele became fascinated with the relationship between food and human settlements. In her well-researched, highly original book *Hungry City,* she explains, through recounting the history of food eaten in London, that food production was once integral in cities and could be again. Before fossil fuels and internal combustion engines, the best way to get meat to the city was on the hoof. Abattoirs within the city—terrible places according to all reports—did the butchering, and the butcher himself was but a few blocks away. Vegetables grew in and close to the city. With fossil fuels, all the messiness, stench, and toil of farming, ranching, and processing food could be banished to the hinterlands. Out of sight, out of mind—and isn't that how it is for us today? If we give credence to peak oil, economy itself says we need to call all those cows and hogs and vegetables back home. Later we'll talk about urban agriculture—the many ways people are growing their own at home in the cities. For now, it's enough to see from the Long Family Farm how close we still are to that way of life. We are food rich compared to many, but the fact is that every road, every parking lot, every skyscraper sits atop soil. It isn't gone. It's just out of sight. And starting to come back to mind.

But when I saw the little meat sign and swerved into the Longs' driveway, I wasn't thinking about all that. I was thinking about red meat, which always brings out a bit of the hunter in me. As I selected my meat from a cooler by a card table under a shade tree, I got to know a few of the Longs. After I paid, Stephani, Leland's wife, took me around to the side of the house to give me one of the slugger bat sized zucchinis stacked on the back porch like firewood—but considerably less useful. As we chatted about the farm I mentioned how much I liked beef liver and tongue, but, with the amount of chemicals fed to factory-farmed animals, I just wouldn't eat them anymore. She disappeared, returning with frozen packages of liver and tongue, which, at that moment, didn't interest their customers. I went home rich in tongue, liver, roasts, hamburger, and enough zucchini for a week. Infused with a disproportionate sense of huntress-prowess, I filled a freezer drawer in my eco-fridge with meat, knowing that in September I would not die from a lack of protein. Plus I'd made back-porch friends with the people who tilled the fields I'd admired as a tourist. I was already eating my way into the heart of the place.

Milk: Telling the Udder Truth

Several years earlier, wanting to expand my repertoire of rural skills, I volunteered as an alternative milker for a friend's goat co-op. At the time I assumed only that it was a lovely way to learn a skill and share some milk.

When I began the hunt for local milk, I asked that friend about her supply.

"Sorry, no can do. You'd have to come and milk the goats yourself because selling milk is illegal. And I'm full up with milkers."

I was confounded. How could anything about milk be illegal? Milk. What about that "Got milk?" campaign where stars wear milk mustaches? Isn't milk like Mother and apple pie?

"It's the raw part," she said. "Unpasteurized milk is illegal to sell."

My first response was to laugh. How ridiculous! But it's true. It is illegal to sell raw milk to the public due to concerns about E. coli, Listeria, and salmonella. Pasteurization handles that for the masses. By heating the milk to below boiling for a few minutes (or up to half an hour, depending on the temperature) and then cooling it rapidly, spoilage slows and thus we can buy "fresh" milk in the grocery store, which lasts for a week in the fridge. Proponents of raw milk say that grass-fed, hygienically handled animals all but eliminate the dangers, but improperly handled raw milk can be a deadly product.

The issues, as you might guess, had something to do with truth (pasteurization does make the nation's milk supply far more safe) and a big something to do with corporate lobbies. More on this later.

Raw milk proponents, though, aren't just Luddites, preferring life in the preindustrial lane. They also claim that raw milk reduces incidence of allergies, asthma, digestive problems, and learning disabilities. It helps with arthritis pain as well as boosting immunity. Some even say it lowers cholesterol and clears cataracts. No wonder my friend sought and found a loophole in the pasteurization laws and started the co-op. She is one of those "The difficult we do today, the impossible takes a little longer" people. No surprise, then, that she found a creative way to obey the law and still have goat milk for the community. If you milk your own goat and drink the milk, it's legal. If you prepare goat cheese from that milk and bring it to a potluck, it's legal. So she gathered a group of sister milkmaids to form a goat co-op. They co-own the herd, take turns milking, buy the feed together, keep records, sterilize their equipment, and provide their co-op members with fresh, delicious milk. When the co-op needed a few backup milkers for vacationing members I got trained, and when called I could take home the absolutely luscious creamy milk. (An aside for those who think "ick" about goat milk: If there are no billy goats around to arouse those sex hormones, goat milk does not taste "goat-y.")

Undeterred, I got the names of people who *do* sell cow's milk out their back door. I can't use their real names, though, which is a pity as they turned out to be so informative, intelligent, and fun. We'll call them Koren and Belinda. I telephoned them and said my goat co-op friend sent me, sort of like "Knock three times and say Joe sent you." Koren said they could supply me with two quarts of milk a week. I'd have to pick it up from the back porch at a set time. I could "rent" the two-quart glass canning jar (they refused to put milk in plastic) if I liked. They'd bill me monthly. Both Koren and Belinda reminded me often that this was a clandestine affair, and over the months gave me an ever-deeper understanding of the issues.

Honey, Cheese, Wine, Coffee & Beans

One person who heard I was committing to a 10-mile diet said, "That should be no problem. You can shop at the Star Store." Yes, the owners are local, but as it turns out, most of the food on their shelves wasn't. I was certain there were beekeepers within my ten miles, though, and I headed down to the Star Store to see if I could find some honey.

I went up and down the aisles, feeling like a stranger in a strange land. To a 10-miler, it was all foreign food. I became like the Ancient Mariner, who when thirsty said, "Water, water everywhere / Nor any drop to drink." Food, food everywhere, but not a morsel to eat. To my relief, there on the shelf was a jar of Island Apiaries honey from Freeland, Washington, less than ten miles as the crow flies. I could be fairly certain the blackberry blossom variety was hyperlocal. Blackberries are outside everyone's back door here. So, sweets: check.

The closest cheese was from Port Townsend on the Olympic Peninsula. Whidbey Island Winery was within my ten miles, but even though they grow grapes there, most of their wines are blends of grapes from other vineyards. And anyway, I am one of those rare birds who get drunk on one drop of wine no matter where the grapes are grown. UBCC (Useless Bay Coffee Company) is catty-corner from the Star Store across Second Street, but they only roast locally. The coffee beans are not Whidbey-grown—not by a long shot.

Speaking of beans, there were dried Rockwell beans in the produce section from Georgie Smith's farm thirty miles north, but none from within my DEZ—designated eating zone. A fourth-generation farmer, Georgie sells her heirloom beans to the Star Store at ten times the cost of ordinary pinto beans, a price only a committed locavore could love (which I became in February when I tried 50-mile eating in the dead of winter—more on that later). Lest you judge Georgie or any local grower as capitalizing on a niche market, overcharging Yuppies with a conscience, wait a few chapters to learn what goes into conventional pricing. The short story—that will get longer as we go on this 10-mile journey together—is that industrial food is cheap because of scale, yes, but also because of subsidies and laws and licensing that favor industrial production. One heretical conclusion I came to is this: we pay too little for food. We do not pay what it costs to produce or what it is worth in scale of importance to us. We also eat far more than we need. You may not agree with me now, or even after reading this book, but stay with me and see how I came to this seemingly unwelcome and inconvenient conclusion before you decide.

There was one 10-mile grower stocking the produce section: Molly Peterson. Her greens, bagged in biodegradable cellophane and labeled with a home-designed sticker, grow less than five miles from my home. In September, though, I'd have all the greens I needed from Tricia. I was looking for what would be missing: meat and sweet. I'd join Molly's Season Extender CSA in October, but for now, her presence was nice but not necessary.

Why Not Fish? You Live Half a Mile from the Beach

I could have eaten clams if I would dig them . . . which was really more effort that I wanted to put out. I didn't eat salmon because I had no access to fish caught within ten miles of my home. Yes, people were pulling them out of the South Whidbey waters by the dozens, but they were probably just passing through. They weren't necessarily 10-mile local, spawned in one of the two salmon creeks on the island. I would have made an exception for Dungeness crab if I could have nabbed one. They creep around in Langley Harbor, probably not scuttling too far afield. Several times I went out in my little kayak and paddled around the dock, looking both hungry and hopeful as people with crab pots returned with their catch.

"Nice big ones!" I'd observe cheerfully.

"Yep."

"Catch a lot?"

"Yep."

"Guess you and your family are going to eat them all, eh?"

"Yep."

"Well . . . enjoy!" I'd say, paddling on, feeling inappropriately deprived. I could have bought a license and pots and caught my own. If this experiment became a post-peak-oil way of life I might, but by then I'd be doing a lot of things differently.

The Four Exotics

I've noticed that as soon as I make a declaration that I will always this or never that, my inner shadow shows up like a film noir character to say, "*Vraiment, chérie? Mais* what about . . . ?" If I make a New Year's resolution to be more kind, the next day my nemesis shows up in full irritating regalia. If I make a resolution to temper my eating, the next day I'm sitting down at a wedding feast.

And so it was that as soon as I accepted Tricia's challenge my mind delivered my list of things I cannot live without and will never find in my ten miles. Even the most dedicated locavores seem to allow themselves a certain number of exotics, foods from outside their eating circle. It's an acknowledgment that fair trading between regions is important, and that life gets a little dull without variety and a few treats. Some choose three foods, some five, some ten. I picked four.

My must-haves were oil (expeller-pressed, of course), lemons and limes, salt plus a few Indian spices, and caffeine. All my exotics are food enhancers, not food itself. They are literally the spice of life. We can live without spice. We can endure anything with concentration and will. But I wasn't about to sacrifice these essentials. Whole continents have been discovered by brave men searching for spices!

Here's my rationale for each one.

Oil is a necessity for preparing food. It gives food color and richness, makes it either crisp or moist, carries flavor, and keeps it from sticking to the pan. You can't stir-fry without oil—or you'll end up with a wok in need of a long soak. Salad dressed with the water it was washed in—that is far too much like dieting. Also, after years of vilifying fats, science now lauds some oils as necessary for heart health—and even sanity (omega-3s have alleviated bipolar illness, according to author Andrew Stoll's research[2]).

Lemons and limes are medicine for me. I attribute the restoration of my liver to good health after my brush with death-by-chemotherapy to a morning glass of hot lemon water, and I drink it daily to this day. I consider it a prescription from my inner doctor. I tried to find a substitute—local apple cider gone to vinegar, perhaps—but didn't find a supplier by September.

Salt and spices provide flavor. I discovered during the month of the challenge that my local herbs—oregano (growing wild in my yard), basil, rosemary, thyme, sage, cilantro, fennel—were lifesavers in making the same veggies daily into different dishes. But salt is food's necessary accessory. Salt is bling. It is glow, glisten, shine, sparkle, depth, passion. Salt, in fact, does not even need to be explained. Yes, in that post-peak-oil scenario I could set up a seawater evaporation system (with sun as the energy source), but I wasn't about to do that for my little 10-mile *month*. This was not about getting an Eagle Scout badge.

Indian spices are another matter. I can't rationalize them except that my hands automatically add cumin, cinnamon, and curry when I cook. My passion for them is supported by more than two millennia of human history. Once Europeans tasted Asian spices they would travel by land and sea at great peril to have them. Perhaps they are even a drug for the taste buds, and if so, I was unwilling to give up my fix. Many studies find them full of healthy phytochemicals and even suggest they moderate blood glucose and reduce inflammation. So perhaps my insistence was my inner doctor again coming to call. Even here, if necessary, I could substitute. Coriander is the seed of cilantro. Fennel, in the celery family, also grows well here and the stalks themselves have a sweet anise flavor.

Caffeine because I need it. I mostly drink black tea and I wasn't giving it up "for all the tea in China." I wasn't about to detox from caffeine along with detoxing from all foods beyond my ten-mile perimeter.

Having negotiated what could breach my dietary walls, I looked more deeply at what else might be necessary to survive the month.

The First Test of My "Yes!"

A few weeks before the starting gun, Tricia called to ask if I liked turnips. I wrote my first blog post:

Tricia brought me some garden "overstock" just before she went to visit in-laws in Iowa. "Do you like turnips?" she asked. Not having eaten them in years I said, "Of course," as this is the response I'm choosing to have whenever Tricia offers me anything. I am going to live almost exclusively from what she grows for the month of September . . . and the turnips are only the beginning.

I can trade what she produces for a few things I just gotta have—milk, honey, vinegar, maybe a chicken or two—but our rule is that these have to come from within 10-miles of our town, Langley, WA. Plus we decided that we can

include 10% "exotics"—tea, salt, oil—as traders have always come through
towns selling spices and teas.

The question is: How local can you go . . . and still have everything you
need . . . and not feel so deprived that you dive into a burger on Day 30.

So about the turnips, I cruised www.recipe.com for some ideas and went with
boiling them in some chicken stock with three onions from her garden and some
garlic left over from Eric's garden (and salt! and spices) and blendered it for an
amazing soup. She'd also given me some kale so I steamed and chopped that and
garnished the soup (well, smothered it) and felt smart, well fed and happy to have
started.

We get going in earnest in September. Meanwhile we are fine-tuning my
10% exotics and our trading partners for the 10-mile extras.

What's the big deal, you might ask. People have homesteads all over the
country. But this is an experiment of a partnership between a market gardener
and a regular person who likes her treats and doesn't grow enough to feed herself
for more than a week a year. It is a community experiment. Not a rugged individual experiment. The bigger question is: in an era of declining energy and other
resources and growing economic instability, in an era when living locally may be
the rule, how well might we manage on our island fare? Can we feed ourselves?
Through our little experiment we are beginning to map the food system in our
community—who has what, how to prepare it, how to trade, how to flourish
where we live.

So to answer the first question: Yes, I like turnips.

Clearly I'd be challenged in many ways this month. I'd eat things I
rarely—if ever—ate, cook in ways I'd never cooked, miss my food
rituals and flavors and habits. Food would not be a backdrop in a
busy life. I wouldn't be able to "grab a bite" and get back to work. For
a month, food would be the main event. I'd spend time washing
and peeling and slicing and chopping and boiling and sautéing and
blendering food. I'd be grateful as never before that I actually had
food to eat.

By August 31 I had it all lined up. Eight pounds of beef in the
freezer. A big jar of honey on the counter. A milk pickup scheduled

for the next evening. Limes from Van's Produce. Plenty of Tetley British blend tea (produced by Tata, the Indian multinational corporation from tea grown on more than one hundred plantations in India and Sri Lanka). And a box of veggies from Tricia in the fridge (more on that in a bit). I gave away to friends everything perishable that was outside my perimeter. Finally, as my last act as a woman free to eat where I could, I took myself out to dinner at the only restaurant within twenty-five miles that served pad Thai. Nice, greasy, noodle-y, peanut-y, chicken-from-a-factory-farm-y pad Thai—my last meal before walking the plank off the ship of food from anywhere and into the murky waters of 10-mile eating.

I got immediate validation from the September 2 Transition Whidbey Potlucks with a Purpose, focused on preparing for their second annual September Eat Local Challenge. Pieces of butcher paper lined the walls of the Fellowship Hall at the Methodist Church labeled meat, cheese, grains, beans, vegetables, fruits, etc. Fifty of us bustled from page to page writing down the island suppliers we'd found for each category. I added some I'd discovered myself, but I was pleased to see that I'd left almost no stone unturned. I'd found just about everything others had found . . . and then some.

One category on the wall that night I hadn't factored in, though, was gleaning. A group called the Gleeful Gleaners had formed at a Potluck with a Purpose the year before. Their goal: to identify fruit trees that went unpicked so the fruit could be harvested and donated to the Good Cheer Food Bank. It was a good reminder that if I couldn't find what I needed from producers in my ten miles, I might find it for free in the forests and abandoned in fields. A group in Bellingham, Small Potatoes had been gleaning for years, bringing in six tons—yes, tons—of produce from local farms and delivering the fruits and vegetables to area food banks, soup kitchens, and feeding programs. They have agreements with more than a dozen local farmers who don't want the food they've grown to go to waste.

Okay, I thought, ready to roll. Bring it on. I'm in. I'm up for it.

Now It's Your Turn

Practice 1: Establish Your Home Base

Whenever you engage in change, you need to know your starting point. What do you eat now?

Start by making a list of the twenty-five (or more) foods you eat most frequently. Not the calories! Not the prices! Not the brands—like McDonald's burgers or Clif Bars! Just the foods. If you can't think of any, just open your fridge and cupboards and see what you have. If you want to be systematic, list foods under the following headings:

Fruits

Vegetables

Meats

Dairy

Nuts

Sweets

Grains

Prepared foods (sauces, mixes, soups)

Practice 2: Your Motivations

In making this personal top twenty-five list, you may become more curious about why you eat what you eat. Why these foods? Why not others? You've seen my hodgepodge list of habits, preferences, ethics, willful denial, addiction, and more. To review:

- Simple: not complex
- Cheap: a bargain
- Healthy: good for me
- Ethical: good for others
- Low-calorie: ain't gonna make me fat
- Desire: I just want it
- Convenience: it's handy

- Comfort: it soothes me
- Nostalgia: what I ate as a kid or at special events
- Because it's there: unconsciousness

Make a list of your own. Ask: Who taught me to like these? Do I eat them from habit or conscious choice? How far do they travel from real food in a field to prepared food on my plate? Who grows and packages and distributes them?

Practice 3: Your Where

You can add a column to your list called "Where?" For each food, write down where it is grown and processed. If you come up blank, treat your industrial food outlet—better known as the grocery store—like a treasure hunt. Bring your list and clipboard and pen and check each food out. If the label doesn't say, ask the produce manager or the store manager. They may not love you for this . . . yet. Later they'll make you the star of their own story of going local.

Food, perhaps more than any other consumer product, is a mirror. Our obsession with diets—health and weight loss—obscures our natural capacity to know what our bodies need. A useful attitude for such inquiry is "no shame, no blame." This is not a new right way. This is you actually beginning to transform your relationship with food—and the hands that feed you.

Practice 4: Begin to Grow Your Own

Growing food used to be a shared endeavor on the part of the whole tribe. To be part of the shift to relational eating—to be part of the tribe—you need to grow at least one crop for home consumption. Fortunately, that's as easy as buying some sprouting seeds and growing them on a windowsill. Sprouting is how you enter relational eating. It's simple, it's inexpensive, and it's a great way to have green food every day—even in winter. Here's how you do it (reading this may take more time than doing it):

Buy some sprouting seeds. You can get them in the bulk section of your store or online. I like the mix with alfalfa, radish, lentil, and others.

Put one to two tablespoons in a wide-mouth jar. There are sets of sprouting lids for mason jars that make rinsing easier, but you can use cheesecloth or muslin and a rubber band to keep it in place.

Fill the jar halfway with water. Put it out of the sun for a day.

Pour off the water through the sieve lid (or remove the muslin), rinse the seeds, pour off that water (replace the muslin if you are using that system), and tilt the jar in a bowl so the water drains.

Repeat whenever you think of it—a couple of times a day.

When the seeds begin to sprout, put the jar in a sunnier spot so the sprouts will eventually green up.

When the jar is full of sprouts and the leaves are green (after four to seven days), you're done.

Rinse them in a big bowl to float off the hulls, then store them in a jar in the fridge. I like to put a paper towel in the jar to absorb extra moisture.

Voilà. You've planted seeds, watered them, and eaten them. Now you're a food producer as well as consumer! That's as local as you can get outside of the bacteria nursery called your intestinal tract.

Ready now to take on more? Anyone who knows me would suggest you look elsewhere for gardening advice, but I know that the best way to learn is on your hands and knees next to a real gardener. Then put a few seeds in the dirt yourself. You can plant in tubs on your balcony or on a patch of yard that you dig up and enrich with compost. Find out from a librarian or farm-and-garden store what grows well in your area so you have success! If you can get a plot in a community garden/pea patch, grab it. Gardening alongside other gardeners is a great way to learn.

Practice 5: Your Food Ethic

Once you have an honest list of what you buy and why, start to think about what conscious criteria you want to put in place. Unfortunately some people who are ethically rigid give "ethics" a bad name. I think of them as steering me toward what I love rather than away from what I fear. I think of them as a beautiful collage I can contemplate to orient me rather than a plaque in the office to say what I have achieved.

Here's a checklist of considerations different people have about the foods they buy and eat. If you believe them all, you might find it hard to shop! If you just buy what you want without any consideration of the effect of the food on your body or other people, you might wonder what the fuss is about. If the list gets you thinking, do some research and make considered choices.

- Price
- How much packaging?
  — None!
  — Nothing you can't recycle
  — BYOB: do you bring your own bag?
  —Don't consider packaging
- Brand
  — Known ethical companies
  — Store brands for price
- How is it produced?
  — Organic
  — All-natural
  — Wild-caught
  — No antibiotics
  — Shade-grown
  — Free range
  — No GMOs (genetically modified organisms)

- Where is it produced?
  — Local
  — Shipped from where?
  — Factory farms?
  — Factory-processed—versus homemade
  — Fair trade?
- What stores—and why
  — Farmers' market
  — Food co-op
  — Locally owned grocery store
  — Chain grocery store
  — Costco/Sam's/Walmart—volume discount stores
  — Online
  — Trader Joe's
  — Specialty stores
  — No stores: gleaning, foraging, freegan (food that is or would be thrown away)
- Where in the store?
  — Produce
  — Bulk bins
  — Only perimeter
  — Which aisles: Frozen? Canned? Boxed? Cereals? Paper/cleaning products?
- Health
  — Raw
  — Cold-pressed
  — No salt
  — No sugar
  — No gluten
  — No nuts
  — No chemicals
  — No meat
  — No dairy

- Religious
  - No pork
  - Kosher
  - No animals
- Ingredients
  - Five or fewer (the Michael Pollan suggestion)
  - No high fructose corn syrup
  - Salt
  - Sugar
  - Colors, flavors, preservatives

Practice Six: Treasure Hunt

Your local farmers and markets are your treasure troves. Use all the tools of the research trade—library, newspapers, Internet, networks, bulletin boards, local food organizations—to find as many of these as you can:

Local farmers' markets
CSAs that serve your area
Good farm stands
Your neighbors' eggs
Food co-ops
Food hubs (resale and distribution points for regional growers)
U-pick berries and vegetables
Pasture-raised beef, chickens, goats, and sheep
Wild-caught fish

Practice Seven: Host a Potluck with a Purpose

Potlucks with a Purpose started right on the front lawn of Island Coffee House in my hometown of Langley, Washington. Our year-old Transition Whidbey group wanted to host enlivening and community-building events that would educate, inspire, inform, and motivate our community. The formula we developed has stood the test of time and traveled to many other Transition groups. Here's the recipe:

A heaping potluck table: best if people incorporate some local foods into their dishes and write the ingredients on a card.

Eating together and socializing.

Celebrations: a moment at the mike for as many as want to for sharing some accomplishment since the last potluck.

Offers and asks: a moment at the mike for as many as possible to offer something they have that they're willing to share or to ask for something they need. Firewood, livestock, furniture, surplus of all sorts, have traded hands through these "offers and asks." One requisite of community is vulnerability, living the truth that we really do need one another. Being able to offer without strings and ask without shame allows resources to flow.

Announcements: a moment at the mike for as many as feasible to announce resilience events. This "town crier" time lets us see how much is afoot.

A connections table: a place where people with offers, asks, and announcements can put their information for others to find it. If a community organization wants to put out information, a member should be sent to make an announcement.

A free box: where people can bring surplus for others to take if they need it—clothes, books, food, toys, whatever.

A meaty, provocative talk or program: a speaker or panel that keeps challenging and informing the community, hopefully to the point of action being taken.

Action groups: existing and newly forming groups meet at the end to plan actions.

Generally, the eating and socializing is a quarter of the evening, the networking is a quarter of the evening, and the program with all the Q&A and action groups is half.

Potlucks with a Purpose promote community without complacency and action without coercion. They are fun events, family-friendly, inclusive. They knit us together by sharing from our surplus and displaying our generous sides. They keep the heartbeat going, feed oxygen to projects, give us courage. They are also like the "welcome wagon" for your community's relocalization efforts. Newcomers can find where to engage or find people to engage with them.

Try These Recipes

Since you've just read about my hunt for 10-mile food, I thought you might like to try a local wild food recipe. Because of the search for local dairy products, Vicky Brown's cheese seems a good piece of knowledge. You'll meet Vicky soon enough; her story of shifting from being a corporate executive to being a milkmaid has many lessons.

Jess Dowdell's Nettle Soup

2 cauliflower heads
3 carrots
3 celery ribs
2 onions
6 Ozette potatoes
½ to 1 gallon stock
½ brown grocery bag full of sweet spring nettle tops (the top 6 inches of the plant)
1 tablespoon minced fresh ginger
Salt and pepper
Crushed red pepper flakes or Mike's hot sauce (optional)

Roughly chop the cauliflower, carrots, celery, onions, and potatoes.
In a large stock pot, sauté the vegetables in local butter or canola oil for about 5 to 8 minutes. Add the nettles and continue sautéing until they are

wilted. Add any kind of stock you wish (I like vegetable or turkey the best) just to cover all the ingredients. Cook on medium heat until the potatoes are soft. Transfer to a food processor or blender, add the ginger, puree, and add salt and pepper to taste. To "heat" it up, add some crushed red pepper or Mike's local hot sauce.

≈

Vicky Brown's Recipe for the Most Simple Dessert of Cheese Makers

The easiest cheese to make goes by many names. It seems that nearly every culture has a version with a different name. It is basic and easy to make with ingredients you have in your home; no ordering cultures from France or enzymes from New England.

This cheese can be made with milk or even whey left from other cheese-making projects. If you're using whey, your yield will be quite small; you might want to add some more milk for a better yield.

For cheese making, never use aluminum. Only use nonreactive pots and utensils (stainless steel, enamel-coated, silicon, and wood are all good options). Heat your milk to about 195°F, stirring constantly to keep it from scalding. Once the heat goes above 192°F add vinegar. I use white vinegar but you could use any type of vinegar. The flavor does not stay with the cheese; you're just using the acidity to coagulate the milk. I've tried it with raspberry vinegar and was very disappointed that the very expensive vinegar did nothing but leave a little pink wash in the curd.

You need to use about ¼ cup of 5 percent acidity vinegar for every gallon of milk or whey. Depending on the starting acidity of your milk or whey you may need more or less. Often people fail at this simple cheese because they stop adding vinegar at the measured amount; just another capful or two might be enough to coagulate your milk.

As you add the vinegar your milk will immediately begin to separate into curds and whey. Once you see the separation make sure your pot is off the heat and let it set for 5 to 10 minutes. The calcium in the curd will cause it to knit together.

You may be able to scoop your curd out of the pot, or you could strain your cheese to separate the curds from the whey and mold it using a colander or basket. Be careful, it is still very hot!

Let the cheese sit about 20 minutes to let more whey drain out, then put it on a plate, sprinkle some cinnamon and nutmeg over it, and drizzle some of your favorite local honey over it. Eat it while it's still warm!

If you prefer savory to sweet you can use it to stuff pasta or mix with herbs or just on a cracker. Once cool enough this cheese could be pressed by hand and refrigerated to make a firm grating cheese. This cheese is also made with any type of milk. Even though I'm partial to my goats and make it often with cow milk, I find that it's heavenly when made with sheep milk!

CHAPTER FOUR

Week One:

Grounded!

Friends and Neighbors

D-Day (10-Mile Diet Day) Minus 1

On August 31, I arrived home dog-tired after a long day in Seattle hauling trash to the dump from my old community house—now on the market. I wanted to eat, which is my basic response to hunger, yes, but also to stress, exhaustion, frustration, and distraction. As well as celebration and excitement. I'd picked up a TJ wrap on the way north, probably the chicken, avocado, blue cheese, lettuce, and mayo one. I had my last bites of industrial food dribbling down my chin as I surveyed the first box of veggies on my counter that Tricia had left, along with a dozen eggs. As of the next morning my life depended on her, and she wanted me to be ready. Beside the box she left this note:

> We did it! After all this talk since July 4 the 10-Mile Diet will start. Yahoo! Here's the first box of veggies and stuff. We can tweak the amount (more or less) as the weeks progress. This should give you a good start. Some things like three turnips and overgrown green beans I threw in hoping you could put them to use. Comments and suggestions will be helpful. My new mantra is freedom and abundance and may we all have it.

The bounty stunned me, like waking up to a mountain of gifts on Christmas morning. Yes, I was a "human subject" for her experiment. But she was volunteering for my experiment as well.

Sure, as Tricia's husband, Kent, later pointed out, from a purely pragmatic perspective, this experiment worked great for frugal me—I was getting free food. But something beyond just "cheap" had started: the bond of love and vulnerability between feeder and eater began with that box of food. Later I came to realize how this experiment was as much about the love as about the food, the knitting together of producer and consumer into the fabric of community. Indeed, one of the oddities, once you think of it, of our modern industrial system is this lack of relationship. I was headed, unknowingly, into relational eating.

Morgan Spurlock's month of McDonald's "super-size me" resulted in a pasty complexion and a bulge over the belt. What would happen during this month of eating Tricia's food, I wondered, as I unpacked that box of turnips, potatoes, onions, green beans, half a head of cabbage, bunches of kale and chard, apples, a big bag of lettuce, pints of cherry tomatoes and strawberries, three Asian pears, three small cukes, and a dozen eggs. Would I become the picture of health? Would I end up hollow-cheeked and as thin as a rail? Would I be able to feel my ribs again? Would I love or hate Tricia for that? I was about to find out.

Nuts!

The first thing that came out of my mouth the first morning of our experiment was "Nuts!" As I shuffled into my kitchen on the first day of this challenge I came face-to-face with the fact that a very cornerstone of my daily well-being—milk for my tea—was missing.

I might even have said something more R-rated, but saying "nuts" here reminds us right off the bat of something else off the menu. Nuts. Normally nuts are a major Vicki food group. They are oily, crunchy, tasty bite-sized packages of perfect pleasure. They go on salads, in stir-fries, in yogurt—and into my mouth morning, noon, and night. Or they did until this morning. Grrr.

Believe me, I tried to find nuts within my 10-mile limits. Walnuts are possible to grow on Whidbey, but I couldn't find any trees. Hazelnuts were a better bet. There was a grove less than a mile from my home that I'd passed through many times on my way to the beach. At least I thought they were hazelnuts, but I'd never really looked closely because before this summer, the natural world was merely backdrop and my food was found not on trees but on shelves.

This grove, however, seemed to have lost the knack of bearing fruit. I remembered that a neighbor had a nut tree—but when I sidled up to him to inquire, I discovered it was for the birds. Literally. He gave up the fight with local wildlife that always picked the tree clean before a single nut could mature. He was quite relaxed about that choice. I wasn't—but it wasn't my tree so I went back to scheming. I asked around and heard about other hazelnut groves, but these were now all squirrel all-you-can-eat restaurants too. To say "nuts" was to remind myself of the great divide that now lay between a favorite food and me.

So, okay, no nuts. But also no milk. Wednesday was my raw milk pickup day—and this was Wednesday—but my milk was still in Elsie's udders. I couldn't get it until seven P.M.

Finding the Treasure in My Own Front Yard

So there I stood, a ratty robe over my cotton nightgown, barely awake yet already bereft. I had hit the twin barriers of food preference and food habit within a half hour of my feet hitting the floor and tucking into fluffy slippers.

The purpose of a chosen constraint like a 10-mile diet is to put awareness above habit and preference. Fasts—be they from overeating, gossip, or chocolate—are essentially reset buttons. They give us a chance to see our inner slob—that creature of lazy routine who prefers never to be upset, challenged, thwarted, or disturbed. The one who sees himself in a magic mirror that takes pounds and years off his body. Who has dozens of excuses about why anything happens (or doesn't), usually starting with "They . . . ," and who can say "I'm awake" quite convincingly in his sleep. Through fasting we poke our sleepy heads up out of the well-worn grooves of our daily lives. We free ourselves one tiny degree further from pride and delusion. But probably not until we've grumbled for a while about it, just as I was doing about the lack of milk for my tea.

I felt like the king in the A. A. Milne poem who wanted "butter for his Royal slice of bread" and was not placated when offered marmalade by the queen instead.

But then I remembered—because creativity blooms when habits and preferences are thwarted—that one day I saw my neighbor Tanya carrying a gallon glass jar of milk into her house. "Bet that was her own bovine contraband!" I called her and, yes, indeed, that had been nectar from Elsie's neighbor Buttercup.

I explained quickly my desperate situation. "Can I borrow a pint of Buttercup's milk? I'll pay you back tonight with Elsie's."

"Sure," she said, and I threw on a coat long enough to hide my bathrobe and nightgown (but still in slippers) and trotted across the cul-de-sac with a clean jar in hand.

I returned home with a satisfying sense of accomplishment. Aaaah! Finally. I had my morning elixir—10,000-mile tea brought to a rolling boil in water from the town well 500 feet away by 100-mile electricity from the Skagit River, sweetened with 10-mile milk and honey. I felt just like the king when he got his butter.

I went out on my deck—journal in one hand, tea in the other—to sit as I did every day, rain, fog, or shine. Today the crystal-white wedge of Mt. Baker shimmered against the blue sky and the waters of Saratoga Passage between Whidbey and Camano Island rested unruffled. Closer in were the village of Langley and Tanya's house across the way. I'd just borrowed the proverbial cup of sugar from her, and by that act I'd crossed the divide between living in a neighborhood and being a neighbor.

A Neighbor in Need . . .

What just happened? I wondered. Yes, I got my milk, clever me, but this warmth in my belly isn't just from the tea. My pen hovered over the page, waiting for this feeling of well-being to translate into thoughts and sentences.

I'm so damned independent. I'm a creature of my country, that's for sure. Live free or die. Well, I guess I almost did. Die, that is.

I crawled onto Whidbey six years ago cut loose by my own choice from all the moorings of my life—a long-standing group household, a home I co-owned, several organizations I was leading. A sane person with stage 3 colon cancer would have stayed where help was always at hand, the rent was free, the food was cooked by others, the meals were convivial, the work was worthwhile and well established, and the networks were strong. But no, I had to go it alone. I thought I did it to face myself, but maybe I was really withdrawing from the pulls and tugs of community. Why else the loneliness?

Moving my weakened body first to Vashon Island, then to Whidbey, brought welcome solitude but unwelcome loneliness—and loneliness revealed a vulnerability I'd never faced before. Activists act. Leaders lead. Now I wasn't the actor in my own movie. I was being "acted upon" by the cancer and by this surprising instinct to encounter myself by myself rather than merely cure myself in the midst of a supportive community.

South Whidbey attracts people in need of quiet, healing, and transition. Its curves are feminine—arcing bays, nubs of hills, round towers of gray clouds that all give the feeling of being swaddled, able to rest. Even back in the wild days when loggers came to turn the island's blanket of cedars and firs into lumber to build the mainland cities, back when Jacob Anthes, Langley's founder, grew tons of vegetables and potatoes for loggers, back when the streets of Langley were muck and mud, women literally ruled the roost. Local historians say that Langley was the first town in the country to elect an all-woman council, shortly after Congress passed the Nineteenth Amendment, giving women the right to vote. Immediately the new mayor, Miss Helen Coe, and her "clean sweep" of councilwomen began civilizing the town.

Just over fifty years later, the town of Langley officially became a city, now inhabited by an influx of hippies as well as conservative Christians, all attracted by the cheap land and mellow way of life. One couple who met and married back then were now my landlords in my small over-the-garage apartment with views of the ragged North Cascades.

Between the time I arrived, paltry possessions in tow, to this "quiet refuge" and the moment I asked for that pint of milk I'd only sipped support from my friends. In my first postdiagnosis year on Vashon I needed them to drive me to doctors' appointments in Seattle. They sat with me during those two rounds of chemo, but once I was dropped off at the Vashon ferry, I was back on my own. New friends on Whidbey, when I had a second surgery, brought me meals for two weeks until I could descend the stairs of my apartment to fend for myself again. Once mobile, I did just that. Fend for myself.

Even after my energy was back and knowledge of peak oil inspired me to start Transition Whidbey with some friends, even after joining a choir and volunteering for a couple of good causes, I was still thinking of myself as a loner.

Until this moment of cul-de-sac neighborliness, though, I didn't recognize the degree to which I still held myself apart here on Whidbey. I engaged in acts of community but not the fact of community. Tanya's easy generosity pierced that protective film of separation. There was no rationale about global conditions or philosophy or morality behind the exchange. I wasn't making something happen self-consciously or courageously. Tanya wasn't bestowing something upon me with beneficence. We were acting as community simply because we were neighbors.

My First Score

At 6.30 P.M., though, you can be sure that I mounted my trusty Europa electric-assist bicycle and pedaled over the highway and through the woods to Belinda and Koren's worn front porch, skirting their pug-faced, super-big, super-friendly dog to get my half-gallon jar of milk from the little fridge by the door. We'd made this agreement only by phone, so making this milk pickup seemed even more furtive. Rich yellow cream floated on the top, a sticky ring clinging to the jar. I hadn't seen top cream like that since the milkman delivered to our back door when I was a child. In those days the glass bottles had a bulb on top where the cream floated so you could pour it off easily. It had been only fifty years or so between that local milkman and these milkers. Less than two generations. In that time there had been a near-tragic disassembly of our local dairies due to rising feed costs even as the price of milk was held steady. My first jug of Elsie's milk gave a glimmer of hope that it might not be too late to restore a more local, low-tech option for dairy.

My young friends Eric and Britt lived not far from Belinda's, and I wanted to see how their gardens were growing. It was late and I'd be riding my bike in the dark if I didn't crank up the throttle on my Europa and speed down the road.

After all of our—okay, my—harebrained schemes of mortgaging ourselves to the hilt to buy a ten-acre ramshackle farm or a hundred-year-old rural church, we'd each settled into more modest and affordable places. They now shared their three-acre Maxwelton Valley property with a flower grower. I wanted to see how their garden was evolving.

By Contrast—Eric's Garden

Eric's permaculture method could not have been more different from my gardening methods carried forward from Rhinelander days. Over tough, established grass he'd laid down manure, then large sheets of cardboard, covering both with straw, and then dug evenly spaced fist-sized holes into the bed, which he filled with compost and vegetable starts. The compost let the plants get established, and by the time the roots reached the manure, it was rotted enough to feed the plant. This was not what we'd figured out in gardening kindergarten, so I wanted to see how it was working. In a word, fantastic.

Eric plans to write a book one day about his method for growing and selling vegetables. He wants to prove that a young person who dreams of farming can, on less than five acres, support himself. When I first met Eric and Britt their dream was a demonstration and education center for sustainability practices. These beds were the beginning of the realization of the dream. I was so impressed but also dismayed. I had seen how minimalist his and Britt's living space was. Was how they lived—home and garden—a model for more than a few courageous sustainability-as-extreme-sport people? My little one-month of minimal food miles seemed tame in comparison, but probably as extreme as I ever wanted to go.

Eric showed me his new setup for taking food to the Tilth farmers' market. He too had a Europa electric bike, to which he hitched a custom-fabricated trailer big enough to haul his week's produce to sell.

"Damn, Eric," I said. "That is so cool. Me, I'd load up my Honda hybrid and consider myself virtuous."

He just smiled in that shy, endearing way that had won Britt's heart and always melted mine. Britt came out in shorts, tank top, and sun hat to woo the ducks into their fenced compound. Between coyotes, hawks, eagles, and raccoons, people on Whidbey shelter their animals at night or lose them (as I had lost my cat Sophie several years before). Besides being literally a farmer's wife, a role she wore gracefully if not willingly, Britt was working for the Sustainable Whidbey Coalition, a network of business and government leaders intent on greening their policies and practices. They snapped her up when she moved on from being executive director of Transition Whidbey.

I met Britt first by phone. My friend Alan had known her in Bellingham and told me she was moving to Whidbey with her sweetheart, Eric—and that we'd love each other. So I called, and I can still remember leaning on the counter in my kitchen, looking out at the mountains and simply "rising" in love with her—her appetite for life, her entrepreneurial drive. It was like meeting a soul sister, and in the years since I've often thought of her as older than me.

I knew she had a big destiny. At twenty-six she seemed like a Great Dane puppy, with doleful eyes, a wiggly body, and huge paws. If you want to know the size of the puppy you are buying, look at the size of his paws. He will grow into them. Britt has, metaphorically speaking, big paws—big work to do. But today, it was the ducks, after which she gave me a hug, and I said good-bye and bicycled home in the waning light.

I thought about them a bit while peddling past the Long Family Farm on Ewing Road.

I had believed in them since my first phone call with Britt even before they landed on Whidbey. But I wasn't convinced—yet—that they could survive on a young farmer's earnings. This troubled me, and made me want to do more research about the economics of farming. These were my friends. This was my community, and I was beginning to see glimmers of what makes local eating a tough row to hoe—so to speak.

By the time I hit the stop sign three miles out of Langley, my bike's electric meter was flickering between yellow and red. I prayed and pedaled my way up the hill, and the e-motor still whirred reassuringly all the way into the garage.

I returned Tanya's milk with interest and then made dinner, which included some goat chèvre from another neighbor.

Cheesy

I'd eaten local goat cheese before, when local goat owners would bring it to potlucks. I found it basically bland and usually went for saltier or sweeter or creamier dishes. In a world where every kind of cheese is available, I would barely label it cheese. More like ricotta, which we all know is edible only as part of goopy lasagna. Okay, so I'm a food snob, but don't we all act as if grocery store shelves spontaneously generate ten thousand food items? Supporting ourselves in the manner to which we've become accustomed requires the whole global production, distribution, and sales system behemoth I'd learn more about as this diet wore on.

Now, though, the thought of goat chèvre was completely intoxicating, so I was thrilled that a peach-perfect teenage beauty, Nina, offered a weekly half-pound tub of her special blend, topped with her trademark pansy. Nina, of course, is not her real name. Not only is dealing fresh-from-the-udder unprocessed goat milk illegal, dealing "value-added" cheese made in uncertified home kitchens is too.

At this point I was willing to be grateful for the cheese and keep my lips buttoned about who made it. Later I would connect the dots and see another piece in the jigsaw puzzle of why local food is expensive and relatively scarce (beyond the three-beet farmers' markets), and why local market gardeners and family farmers are battling their way into the marketplace against a tidal current of industrial food.

I'd met Nina when she was a thin shadow trailing after her strong-minded mother, Sandra. Now she was ripening into a young woman. She and her folks, Sandra and Hal, have a little homestead out toward Clinton where Nina loves making cheese from the family's extra goat milk.

Nina found out about my 10-mile diet from the crackling grapevine here on South Whidbey. Whidbey is fundamentally a rural community where word of mouth is still the most efficient medium of communication. Nina, perhaps with Sandra's prompting, stepped forward. And for the month of the experiment she chose to put a gift cardboard tub by the door each week for me to pick up.

Hometown Cooking

As I scooped a few teaspoons of chèvre onto my stir-fry that evening, I reflected on how the generosity being served along with the food I was eating—Tricia's and Nina's food, Tanya's milk loan—gave a new meaning to *home cooking*. I was cooking food from my hometown as well as cooking food in my home. Not only that—these people were treating me like family.

We don't charge our families for dinner. We contribute to the common family good out of some blend of love and duty, but not for money. I call that our "circle of we," those we consider our own, our kin. We are living in a time when the bonds of family are looser than ever, when children live far from parents, where our "communities" might be online, not next door, where—as Robert Putnam called this alienation in his book *Bowling Alone*—we now "bowl alone," not together in leagues. We have lost a sense of community. It is a great feeling to receive care just because I am there. I relished this budding sense of belonging to others through my 10-mile experiment as I salted my meal, wishing for soy sauce but happy anyway.

It seemed to me that in those idealized bygone eras, people shared their plenty freely. I wondered about what was now not just "the" island but my island, so after dinner I pulled out Lorna Cherry's two-volume local history, *South Whidbey and Its People*. The first volume was actually typewritten double-spaced! The second was typeset but still clearly homegrown. I'd gotten them when I first arrived and read through with the curiosity of a tourist. Now I wanted to know what my people ate fifty to one hundred years ago.

Island of Plenty

In the first volume Lorna reports an abundance of food when the first settlers arrived: berries grew everywhere. Deer, bear, elk, wolves, squirrels, mink, otter, weasels, raccoons, beaver, rabbits, and foxes lived in the dense old-growth forests. In the open fields and along the shores, ducks, geese, grouse, and pheasants made homes. The sea too offered huge bounty—clams, crabs, mussels and clams, halibut, herring, flounder, octopi, and, of course, salmon.

The plenty bred a spirit of generosity in the Coastal Indians who camped here in the summer. The potlatch started in the Northwest—the gifting ceremonies where the powerful could share their bounty with the poor because hoarding in a land of plenty made no sense.

In nature, plants store but do not hoard. They grow thick roots to store sunlight. They grow storage vessels—husks and fruits and shells—to protect seeds. But in nature, hoarding throws ecosystems out of balance.

Once, sitting next to a tree in the Amazon rainforest, I seemed to hear it tell me: "Everything in the community of life gives back to life 100 percent—except the humans. We are the species that hoards." The novelist Daniel Quinn in his award-winning novel *Ishmael* calls us—the people who enter the lands of others to confiscate their resources—the "takers." A century ago, settlers on Whidbey took these lands as their own, displacing the tribes who had roamed here, feeding on the plenty.

Lorna's second volume about Whidbey documents these years of growth and development. South Whidbey, where I live, had thinner, rocky soil. To this day gardeners pull out rocks along with weeds year in and year out as ever more of the glacial till flows to the surface. Farther north, though, where the island is nipped in as if by a corset and the land lies low, farmland with topsoil several feet deep drew the early settlers to edge out the natives (with some violence on both sides) to grow wheat. No wonder that in 1919 Whidbey captured first, second, and third prizes in the national wheat contest in Philadelphia. Whidbey had the world record—117.5 bushels of wheat per acre! Island County promoted itself to new settlers with a pamphlet called *Whidbey Island, World Beater*—because of our wheat. In the late 1930s an article in the *Whidbey Record* proclaimed, "Whidbey Is the Best Farm Locality In the World; Climate, Soil, Markets, Best Suited For Agriculture."

In the century between then and now Whidbey had gone through similar transformations to those across the United States—a slow shift from rural to urban, from homegrown to industrial-grown, and from large families to small to many choosing the single life. The

"World Beater" title would sooner go to a big box store than a wheat crop.

A century ago 66 percent of all households in the United States had more than five people.[1] In 1930, 25 percent of the U.S. population lived on 6 million family farms.[2] Farming families were a built-in circle of we. Sharing was the unquestioned norm. When did we change? Why do nearly a third of us now live alone in tight little circles of me, myself, and I?

As noted earlier, some say that the longest journey in the world is the soul's twelve-inch migration from head to heart. Culturally I believe the long walk to new patterns of sanity, security, safety, wealth, and happiness will be on a road called "from me to we." In the years ahead it will be natural for ever more of us to metaphorically put on our robes and slippers and trot across the cul-de-sac from our "single person living alone" status and join at least with neighbors, if not with housemates, husbands, or entire blended families.

Just a Bite Before Bed—Not

It was late by then. I had read and mused for several hours and was ready for bed. More like ready for one more eating hurdle. The bedtime snack. Or, more honestly put: the bedtime minigorge. Ask me my favorite position and I'd have to say, "Facing an open fridge in the dead of night, spoon in hand."

Grrr. The NPD (formerly National Purchase Diary) Consumer Research Group issued a report in 2008 called *Snacking in America*.[3] In it they called snacking "the fourth meal of the day." For my other three meals in the days ahead I was able to eat frittatas in the morning, salads at noon, and stir-fries at night and wax poetic or at least self-congratulatory about the experience. Now I was facing despair and deprivation.

How could I shovel any of this food—grown, and given with love—into my mouth like a pacifier? The desire for crunch, for volume, for bending my elbow in service to my mouth, met the commitment to an experiment in hyperlocal eating. Overeating isn't just abusing my body. Now it is abusing my farmers. Wandering Tricia's garden, watching her pull stray weeds and tuck tomato vines back into their wire supports, you can't think of her food as merely fodder for her bank account. It is her love making vegetables sweet. And I'm going to eat all the snap peas in a five-minute orgy of chewing? I don't think so.

The only parts of me that went to bed satisfied that night were my virtue and wisdom. I lay down with my grrring mind and growling stomach flouncing around petulantly and soothed them with "It's only a month."

That world-beater wheat was a century in the past. Any grain, in fact, was a month in the future, since it all grew up there on the prairie, twenty-five miles as the crow flies from my mouth. I felt like a poor kid on a December night—her face pressed against the plate-glass display window at FAO Schwarz with the finest toys in New York inches away, solidly out of reach.

What's Local

That Saturday I went to the Bayview farmers' market to see what else I might find—whether farmers to chat with or 10-mile treats.

Like so many farmers' markets, the Bayview one sprouts each Saturday like mushrooms after rain—a full-blown festival of food, crafts, and music in a parking lot. Ours is between the old Bayview Community Hall and the old Cash Store, renovated to a high-sustainability standard to house shops, offices, and a restaurant. It's been hallowed community ground for a century.

There you'll find Dorcas and her son James selling spicy African food and vegetables, plus there's often kettle corn, barbecue, and tastes of cheese from Vicky Brown, bread from Tree Top Bakers, and a paper cup with a bit of brown rice topped with Mr. Mobley's irresistible secret-recipe sauce, served by Neal Mobley himself. You can get fresh-cut flowers, fresh-spun yarn, and to-die-for pies. Oh, and lots of vegetables from island farms.

At Bayview I stopped to chat with Pam Mitchell, the systematic market gardener who spoke at our first Transition Whidbey potluck. She'd sold at the farmers' market there for more than a decade, and for a few years had been the market manager, setting and enforcing parameters for who can sell what. A persistent debate runs about how far afield, so to speak, the produce can grow. Must it be the island? The four-county region (Skagit, Whatcom, Island, Jefferson)? What about east of the Cascades, where warm-weather crops flourish? Can that be considered local?

According to the USDA, yes. Local means four hundred miles from source to store:

> Though "local" has a geographic connotation, there is no consensus on a definition in terms of the distance between production and consumption. Definitions related to geographic distance between production and sales vary by regions, companies, consumers, and local food markets. According to the definition adopted by the U.S. Congress in the 2008 Food, Conservation, and Energy Act, the total distance that a product can be transported and still be considered a "locally or regionally produced agricultural food product" is less than 400 miles from its origin, or within the State in which it is produced.[4]

To a 10-miler, of course, 400 miles sounds ridiculous—so bosomy as to not even fit into any tidy understanding of this "local" value. But that number later would take on a world of meaning for me.

At Bayview, though, local is, well, more local. Island growers are given a comparative advantage by rewarding them with prime "real estate" for their stalls. Pam's seniority, for example, has netted her a spot on the outer rim of the market, in the shade, between the two most used entrances. This is one of the hundreds of microissues along the border between anywhere food and local food. Tomatoes, for example, are simply more challenging to grow here than in the sunny fertile fields of eastern Washington. Calling both local and selling them side by side makes survival for our island growers just that much more precarious. Even here in this little corner of the earth the trade issues debated in global fora show up. Where are the borders? What "market rules" will protect the little guy without punishing those who've figured out how to scale up? Viable regional food systems are critical if more of us are to eat more food grown closer to home, but how to support regional systems, and especially the local growers, will have to be figured out one transaction, one decision, one conversation, at a time.

I've shopped farmers' markets since the first one sprouted in a community center parking lot in Seattle in 1993. A few years earlier we'd signed on with the first CSA in the region, Helsing Farm in Chehalis, Washington. Even so, I'd never understood, as I now do because Pam and others explained it, the blood, sweat, tears, and a thousand decisions that go into those seamless Saturday shopping experiences.

Pam Mitchell

Pam is the picture of a local farmer—round ruddy cheeks, slightly eccentric style, fingernails rimmed with permanent dirt.

Pam's signature look is her bowler hat, always tilted back on her head atop a fringe of strawberry-blond bangs that frame her face. She is no central-casting rube, though. Her eyes are intelligent, as are her strategies for making a living farming. Pam works late into the evening the day before the market, harvesting the week's produce, cleaning and bagging it, packing it into bins that then slide into her truck, ready for the wee-hour transfer to her Bayview stand. Depending on the season, Pam has vegetable starts (you can buy enough starts for a whole garden for a reduced price). She has biodegradable bags of salad greens and basil and net bags of squash, green beans, eggplant, potatoes, and garlic. She'll have mountains of tomatoes and whatever variety her plots are producing

Pam knows—to the penny—what it takes to support herself as a market gardener. She knows what sells, what each bed in her garden yields, what her year-over-year growth is, and what the net is for her selling at the flourishing farmers' market across the water in Everett (counting gas and time) versus the less-frequented Sunday Market at Greenbank Farm. This is not an experiment for her. It's her life.

Her farming life, in fact, began when she was two and helped her paternal grandfather in the family garden in Cape Town, South Africa, where she grew up. Her mother reported that she'd watch Pam out the window eating soil (very good for the immune system). Farming literally got into her blood early in life, and she naturally became the family farmer and then got her horticultural degree in Cape Town, preparing for a lifetime of growing food. Reality struck. Making living things grow didn't add up to making a living. She worked for years in the corporate world but, through will and grit, ultimately landed that "sharecropping" situation on the property of a high-end catering company on Whidbey, achieving a rarity: a farmer without a mortgage.

She'd dreamed all along that one day she'd kiss the corporate world good-bye. Now she'd done just that. More than marriage, more than family, more than fame and fortune, Pam derives her joy, satisfaction, and identity from farming.

The more I got to know Pam during and after my 10-mile diet, the clearer it became that I had asked the perfect person to give our Transition Whidbey community its first taste of how bare our larders would be if for some reason we needed to depend—all of us—on what we could grow here. As you recall, she did a rough calculation of population, land in production, and crops we can currently grow in the summer season. Her conclusion was that if all sixty thousand island residents had to depend on what our 170 square miles—less than 15 percent of that in farmland—could produce, we'd survive a month, that month being August. As Whidbey is mostly rural, I'd bet dollars to doughnuts (which were also missing in my 10-mile diet) that the 200 square miles around you would be no better and maybe far worse than Whidbey in feeding her folk.

Manna from Heaven

On my way home from the market I swung by the middle school football field, where Kent was announcing a Little League game and Tricia was running the scoreboard. She had told me to come by and pick up some veggies that were a bit too big or curly or twisty for her regular customers. I stood under the viewing box, elevated twenty feet to observe the whole playing field, so I could catch a bag from her and bicycle home. Here were two acts of community: Kent with no skin in the game (no kids on the field) was giving his time just because he is part of this place; Tricia simply gifted me.

As I rode home the word *natural* came to mind because this easy give-and-take among people in community felt natural. Back when I lived in intentional communities the flow of stuff and services was the most natural thing—an endless river of hand-me-ups and -downs. Though I live more conventionally now, my native habitat is sharing. Until this 10-mile experiment I'd felt a bit like a fish out of water. I breathed in a money atmosphere. Most people and even time itself were busy—dammed, clogged, not flowing freely. Now I was bathing in community again—and it felt natural.

The word *natural* when used with *food* has no official meaning. Products are labeled "natural" and we think that means straight from the source—land, sea, or air—containing no additives and minimally processed. In the United States, however, there are no firm standards for this assertion. The term also says nothing about our relationship with food—about either our fear of tainted food from afar or our longing for wholesome food to feed ourselves and our families.

My 10-mile diet, by taking out the middlemen—the packagers and distributors and shippers and grocers—was putting verifiably unprocessed natural food into my belly, but it was also doing this other thing, this relationship thing. I could literally feel the love, not just presume it because of a label or standard or picture on a carton. I could touch not just the food but my feeder—and damn if it didn't feel good.

So as I glided into my garage, plugged my bike in to feed it some electrons, and lifted the bag of baroque green beans, squash, and potatoes out of the pannier, I decided to call my relationships with Sandra, Tricia, Pam, and Nina "natural food." Perhaps soul food is just this: that food given to us by people we know—as gifts, as dinner—feeds the soul.

Steamed veggies never tasted so good.

Tally—Week One

Just before Tricia delivered her second box I tallied my intake on my blog:

> I've eaten through three turnips, five potatoes, three onions, half a garlic head, bunches of kale and chard, 11 eggs, a quart of milk, a pint of cherry tomatoes, a pint of strawberries, two apples and three Asian pears, a big bag of lettuce, three cuke-ettes, a small bag of basil, one pound of Long Family beef, raw honey from Island Apiaries, a few snow peas, leftover chicken from Britt and Eric's wedding, those green beans—plus from my garden I've gotten three carrots, four cukes, some kale, some oregano and a bowl of green beans. From the roadside I picked a pint of blackberries and nary a scratch as I was out there with my protective clothing, clippers and a hoe (yes, these are killer berries). From my neighbor's daughter I got goat cheese that I'm still working on. And I don't know what I would have done without my exotics: oil, tea/coffee, lemons and salt.
>
> I think that's it. Sobering really to both see how much I eat and how vulnerable I am to Tricia continuing to produce enough.
>
> Ready for week two.

Now It's Your Turn

Location, Location, Location

Are you planted where you want to bloom? "Location, location, location" is a real estate mantra for purchasing a home: views, schools, economy, culture. From a local food perspective, location refers to climate, soils, sun, wind, and water.

Bloom where you are planted is best. Adapt your home and community to the changes ahead. The social, cultural, and relational wealth you've built where you now live are crucial for survival of both body and soul. The grass may look greener elsewhere, but, as Erma Bombeck once pointed out, it could be because it's over the septic tank. You do want to take an objective look at your home, though, to see if the disruption of moving is offset by the benefits. Begin researching:

- What did people here eat two hundred years ago? One hundred years ago?
- What fruits and vegetables grow well here?
- What might the weather be fifty years from now?
- Where does the water come from?
- What is the solar, wind, geothermal, and water potential of this property—even if it is in the middle of a city?

Visit your local farmers' market with an eye to understanding the whole operation, not just buying a few beets. Within a few years you should find somewhere you care about and live a life that shows it!

Try These Recipes

Because soup is such a staple of a local diet, I thought you'd like to know how Jess Dowdell makes stock. I'm also including Jess's recipe for lamb, because, as I discovered later, it's also a great way to cook a leg of goat.

Basic Vegetable Stock

Jess says:

I love to make stock with the vegetable trims from the kitchen. I think of stock as the essence of the kitchen, if you will, a story of the season, the farm, the harvest, and the creation. So it's always good to start with food that is not grown with pesticides, herbicides, or hormones and ones that are genetically modified. I try to source all food locally, organically, and sustainably grown. I feel that when I know the farmer, then I know the story. Stock is nutritious and delicious just as it is or added to other creations. By keeping a container in the refrigerator to collect trims, nubs, and misfits that have already been washed your work is almost done! In my stock I like a balance of flavors that can be used to add complexity to any soup, sauce, cooking broth, or whatever, depending on the menu. I've been known for a few odd combos, but they are always fun and tasty. One time I put coffee in my stock (I love Caffé Vita from Seattle) and it actually worked! I used the "coffee stock" to braise Whidbey-pasture-raised lamb shanks, then later added red wine from Whidbey Island Winery, and, finally, just a touch of hot peppers from Bur Oak farm stand. What a wonderful treat. Anyway, this list is loose and free for the season and mood to dictate. It doesn't hurt to play with different combinations. It's compost otherwise, right?

Using a large stock pot, I always start with onion, carrot, celery, and herbs of any kind, and add any combination of the following, bring to a slow simmer, and let barely simmer for as long as 3 to 4 hours. Periodically skim off the foam as it rises to the top of your pot. I've gone longer on bone marrow stock, cooking it from 8 to 24 hours.

When finished cooking, strain the broth, and now your stock is ready for use or for the freezer. Have fun!

Veggies

Snap peas

Snow peas

Beets and greens

Chard

Corncobs

Kohlrabi

Kale: lots of different kinds (peacock-flowering)

Shallots

Spring greens

Dandelion greens

Green onions

Garlic

Melon rind

Peppers (hot—jalapeño, Scotch bonnet, cayenne—is good but any
will do)

Parsnip

Any potatoes

Zucchini/squash

Tomatoes

Turnips

Herbs

Basil

Dill

Oregano

Tarragon

Cilantro

Parsley

Any others that you already have

Feel free to add meat bones, cooked or raw, to make protein stocks.
Same principle!

Jess's Coffee and Red Wine–Infused Lamb

2 tablespoons vegetable oil

3 lamb riblets or lamb shanks (locally grown)

Salt and pepper

2 teaspoons crushed red pepper (or more for spicier meat)

1 small red bell pepper, chopped

1 large onion, chopped

3 garlic cloves, chopped

2 dried pasilla chile peppers, stemmed, seeded, and minced

1 cup red wine (from Whidbey Island Winery)

1 cup strong coffee (I love Caffé Vita)

Preheat the oven to 350°F.

In a heavy cast-iron pot that can later be covered, drizzle oil and brown the lamb on all sides over high heat. Season with salt and pepper to taste and crushed red pepper as it cooks. Remove the lamb from the pan and lower the heat to medium. Cook the pepper, onion, garlic, and chiles in the pan, stirring occasionally, about 10 minutes, until the onions and peppers are soft. Add the wine and coffee and reduce the heat by about half. Return the lamb to the pot, cover, and cook in the preheated oven for 2 to 3 hours. Turn the meat a few times while it's baking. Pull all the meat off the bone and serve hot.

CHAPTER FIVE

Week Two:

Getting the Hang of It

The warm fuzzies I was getting from this diet were great, and my body felt healthier than ever, but there was still something missing from my life—CRUNCH. And this set me off, surprisingly, on a hunt for more zucchini, which led to lessons in a new kind of cooking in my kitchen and a mystical experience in my backyard. Let's start with the zucchinis.

The joke around here is that in September, *no one* hunts for zucchini—in fact, you need to lock your door to keep neighbors from depositing oversized black beauties in your house while you sleep.

BTD—before 10-mile diet—I'd have taken such precautions. In fact, I have foisted zucchinis on whoever would take them. Now that I found myself stalking the elusive crunch, though, I was vulnerable to anyone's cockamamie ideas for crunch. I forget who told me I could turn zucchini into crispy chips. I didn't know if they were sniggering in the bushes and sending me on a wild goose chase (hmmm, wild geese, I wonder . . .). It didn't matter. I was desperate. With visions of corn chips and potato chips dancing in my mind, I followed their instructions.

Zackers

I want to first draw your attention to the how of this story as well as the what, because how I made those first zackers (zucchini crackers) is important, no matter what the results.

In my first year on Whidbey I bought a countertop convection oven at the thrift store simply to save energy now that I was just cooking for one. It had a mysterious DEH setting. It never occurred to me that DEH stood for "dehydrate" or that I'd someday need this feature. But when a new-in-the-box set of dehydrating racks later showed up at the thrift store for this very oven, something told me I should buy them. I had no intention of spending my life energy slicing and drying fruits and veggies, but you never know (a phrase that's the hallmark of a true thrift-store junkie). The "recovery" could turn into a nasty recession again and I'd be protected by . . . dehydrating racks. The logic isn't perfect, but at least my 10-mile diet vindicated the choice.

Due to my early years living off the land and on the road, living on one hundred dollars a month, I host an inner survivalist who never sleeps, who prowls the thrift store keen for castoffs for my stash. I've stocked my shed with survival essentials from the thrift store: a new-in-the-box Mexican hand grinder (for corn tortillas), canning jars and lids, pressure canner, machete, bow saw, hand tools including a hand drill Joe Dominguez bought with his birthday money when he was seven in 1945. I pray that I'll never have to use any of them. I don't relish the thought of limited electricity. I am not rooting for the demise of Western civilization. Nonetheless, I value the products of all human evolution up until pretty much the post–World War II rise of small electric appliances. Even my dehydrator could be replaced by the sun, but the need for crunch—now!—meant I needed local electrons to help me out.

The recipe sounded easy: just slice the zucchini into quarter-inch-thick rounds, fill the racks, pop them in the convection oven at 125 to 145 degrees, and remove them when the chips are crisp but not burned. Aah, crisp. Even the word makes me salivate. Toasted sourdough French bread. Dry-roasted nuts. Fresh rye crisp. Tortilla chips dipped in hot sauce, piled high in Mexican restaurants while you peruse the menu. Chitlins. Crunch! Not until this diet confronted me with the absence of my daily crunch did I have to face this addiction.

Crunchaholics

Am I alone in this? Apparently not. Psychologists like Linda Spangle are making names for themselves by identifying the difference between people like me—crunchies—and chocoholic sweeties. Crunchies have what she calls "head hunger." We are, according to Linda, stressed and irritated, which is about how I feel when I don't have crunch. Her point exactly. Sweeties are sad and lonely. Linda calls theirs a "heart hunger." Clearly that is a secondary need for me—otherwise I would have insisted on chocolate as exotic number five.

Such psychological displacement isn't bad—none of us is a saint. Better chocolate bars than singles bars, better crackers than crack.

To verify how "crunchy" Americans really are, one needs only to peruse the cereal aisle at the grocery store. The elder of the aisle is Kellogg's Rice Krispies, a hit from the day they were released in 1928 with their signature "snap, crackle, and pop." Cheerios have always been crunchy, but now we have Cheerios Crunch as well. There's a crunch for every occasion—and taste: Cap'n Crunch, caramel Crunchfuls, Sun Crunchers, Cruncheroos, Go Lean Crunch!, and even Krusty-O's, which might satisfy the ever-bumbling Homer Simpson's need for crunch.

Just in case this house of cardboard cereal boxes comes down, though, won't we all be glad to know about zackers?

Right from the oven, on the edge of burned, zackers do the crunch trick, especially with enough salt. Store in an airtight jar to distribute the crispiness evenly, and they may even retain some jaw-delighting snap. Even if/when they devolve from crunchy to chewy, according to Linda Spangle, our jaws will get the grinding we need. No wonder "something to chew on" means something to think about. We heady crunchies love that.

When my zackers didn't quite satisfy, I found a slather of local butter along with the salt helped.

Butter for the Royal Slice of . . . Zacker

Butter? That wasn't on the local list, but when I complained to a friend about the lack of "butter for the Royal slice of . . . zacker," she said I could have it in two—or more—shakes.

"Don't you know, you can make butter out of your raw cream?"

"No way."

"Way." Which could also be spelled *whey*, which is what's left once the butter is churned.

She explained the basic technique, apparently taught to all second graders except me. You put cream in a jar and then shake it vigorously until a ball of butter magically appears in the thin grayish whey.

If you are my age, I suggest wearing a snug long-sleeved jersey—or support hose up to your armpits—so your upper-arm wattle won't jiggle the entire ten minutes needed to coax the butter out of the cream. If you are a member of a gym, this activity might save you the monthly fee, especially if you jiggle and jog at the same time.

For me it was so worth the effort. The butter was okay, but demystifying butter was even better. I remembered that in the "olden days" women churned butter. I'd even seen women in bonnets and long calico dresses do it in reenactments of Colonial life in Williamsburg, Virginia. However, I simply made no connection between that quaint tableau and my current life, where butter comes in wax-paper-wrapped cubes. Until I saw the proof that butter requires only cream, a jar, and some upper-body endurance.

When I wanted something like a cookie—creamy, sweet, and crunchy—I just put some local honey on a buttered zacker. Voilà! A zookie. I was like Tom Sawyer, so convincing about the pleasures of zackers and zookies that everyone wanted to try them. Watching their faces as they chewed away at my leathery treasure, I realized that these Zookies and Zackers were not necessarily the best advertising for a 10-mile diet.

Cooking from Scratch

Cream wasn't the only "ingredient" I had to turn into food. None of my 10-mile foods came with recipes. None had nutritional labeling so that I could calculate my protein and vitamins for the day. Some I'd never even eaten before. Remember, in August I had to turn to recipes.com to find out what to do with a turnip.

As September rolled on, though, I found that site and my half-dozen stalwart cookbooks less and less helpful. I couldn't really use them as written. I was missing too many ingredients. In the absence of capers, anchovies, flour, sugar, baking soda, baking powder, rice, wheat, corn, noodles, nuts and nut butters, creamed canned soups, and on and on, I was thrown back on my own resources.

What I reclaimed when I let go, though, was resourcefulness. I was learning to cook without recipes the way you learn to ride a bicycle without training wheels or ice skate without gripping the side railing and mincing around the rink.

I learned how to address a zucchini—as well as kale, chard, beans, snow peas, basil, oregano, potatoes, beets, carrots, onions, garlic, kohlrabi, rutabagas, turnips, and did I mention kale?—the way a karate master might address a plank he was going to break with his bare hands. Utter attention, respect, and presence. I needed to listen to what the zucchini—or any food—could become.

Slowly I shifted from seeing my range of ingredients from limited to limitless, from a few dozen ingredients to endless possibilities for delicious meals.

Take zucchini—just to pick a vegetable randomly out of a hat. Not only did I roast or bake or dehydrate it in my convection oven, I sliced it into wedges lengthwise like cucumber sticks. I used a serrated peeler that produced long strands of "zukett." I julienned it (more to come on this method) for stir-fry, I lightly steamed chunks, which I could eat as a side vegetable or blend into soup with some garden herbs.

Or take kale, my other fail-safe crop. It can be steamed, dehydrated, stir-fried, and added to soups. Baby kale can go into salads raw. Curly kale can cup potato salad on a platter to make that pot-luck dish look "dishier." Best of all, kale can also make kale crisps.

Green beans can be pickled as well as steamed, fried, added to soups, or crunched (aah, that blessed word!) raw as you walk bare-foot in the morning through the dew in the garden.

Beets can be shredded onto salads, roasted, made into pickles, made into borscht, or just boiled. The leftover water can be used to make beet wine (which we did in Rhinelander under the tutelage of the Lithuanian neighbors, ending up with something akin to decent port). On those long winter subzero nights, when playing cards or end-less philosophizing weren't enough to see us through the boredom, that beet wine tempered those tempers that cabin fever can ignite.

And God, the potato! What can't you do with a potato? You can bake it, fry it in thin rounds to be chips or in sticks to be "freedom fries," or slice it a bit thicker for a frittata. You can shred it for fritters, boil it for mashed potatoes, or blender it for a creamier soup. Not only that, but it's a lifesaver. You can chunk potatoes as a correction for an oversalted stew or soup. The neutral, generous potatoes will mop up the excess and balance the pot.

Apples as ingredients are simply amazing. You can eat them, of course. But you can cook them down into applesauce and further down into apple butter. You can bake them with some honey, cinna-mon, and nutmeg dribbled down the core. You can also slice and de-hydrate them for a chewy snack later. If you juice your veggies, apples can be thrown in after kale and beets to make the slurry actu-ally palatable. They bring sweet and tart. They bring crisp. They bring color when chopped into a salad.

Each fruit, each vegetable, can be used for its many qualities: color, texture, where it sits on the sweet-to-sour scale, how it trans-forms when cooked. They aren't just "called for" in someone else's recipe. If you approach them with curiosity and amazement, you can hear them telling you what to do.

Sugar and Spice and Everything Nice

One thing you'll learn right away if you ever attempt your own version of a 10-mile diet: herbs and spices are crucial to cooking from scratch.

I really got it why women of yore had herb gardens—and vegetable gardeners these days do too. Take that zucchini. It's one thing with basil, another with rosemary, another with garlic, yet another with oregano. Herbs relieve the monotony of a simple diet.

It never occurred to me before that herbs and spices are different. They shared shelf space in the store and the same greasy rack on my kitchen counter, and that was that. Now, hungry for any crumb of wisdom, I almost snorted whatever knowledge I found. Sometime during week two, I spotted a fat volume called the *Dictionary of Food* in a used-book store and snapped it up. I bought it, brought it home, and for the rest of the month it sat on my kitchen counter so I could peruse it daily. Every page was an eye-opener! Who knew there were fundamental differences between herbs and spices? Herbs come from, duh-uh, leaves of herbaceous (nonwoody) plants. Spices come from the roots (ginger), flowers (cloves), fruits (vanilla), seed (cumin), and bark (cinnamon) of plants. I felt like I was in grade school in the daily wonder of discovery. Further, I learned that herbs are generally European in origin and spices are from tropical climates. This is why herbs were a slam dunk on a 10-mile diet and spices were not. They have to squeak in under the term "exotics." Another duh-uh.

Along with the "real" food, i.e., what I could actually chew, Tricia's boxes came with bags of parsley, sage, rosemary, and thyme. Another duh-uh. Could this be why Simon and Garfunkel's rendition of "Scarborough Fair" had these herbs in the refrain? Was it because these flavors—now essential for adding interest to my veggies—were long ago essential for turning medieval slop into tasty dishes? Further, did they have a function in keeping us well?

A study by the Nutrition Research Institute[1] project director and University of North Carolina professor Martin Kohlmeier, M.D., reveals why I, a lowly consumer, was not informed about the medicinal properties of food. In the study, 109 medical schools were surveyed and only 28 of them met the National Academy of Science requirement of even twenty-five hours of nutrition education.[2]

I was certainly a poster child for the failure of our medical system to educate us on that food/medicine link. My diet was waking me up, though. Herbs and spices are used not just in cooking but in healing. All medicines once originated in nature. Where else would they come from?

We think of medicines as pills in jars, not leaves and seeds and bark and flowers. It's obvious, but until that moment I'd never put it together. When I quit chemo the naturopath prescribed turmeric— the same spice that's in curry. Reading up on this spice/medicine, I found it's even used to *prevent* cancer!

Only now is the food industry touting "functional foods"—ones with some smidgen of health-promoting, disease-preventing, or healing properties. What could be more functional, though, than fruits and vegetables—the mainstay of my 10-mile diet?

When Hippocrates said "Let your food be your medicine and your medicine be your food," he must have meant just what I was discovering as I read the *Dictionary of Food*.

Tools of the Trade

The final "ingredient" in my 10-mile kitchen was my stash of simple cooking tools.

I already mentioned the convection oven. In addition to producing zackers, it also did a fine job of roasting zucchinis sliced the long way, like chicken fillets, slathered in oil, and salted. The bigger zucchinis could be baked almost like winter squash—seeds scooped out and the cavity filled with sautéed chopped carrots, eggplant, and even Long Family beef. The oven was even big enough to roast a chicken, which I did as a treat at the end of the month.

The convection oven was one of my top eleven tools for turning the bounty in my yard and fridge into breakfast, lunch, and dinner and those minimeals in between. The others were

- a chef's knife
- a 4-quart pot with a steamer basket
- a heavy 8-quart pot
- a pressure cooker/canner
- a cast-iron skillet
- a mandoline
- a Zyliss slicer
- a food mill
- a peeler
- a blender

Perhaps I should have gotten a food processor and become Martha Stewart–proficient with it. That didn't occur to me. For one thing, the thrift store never had one, and I treat the thrift store as an angel of God—answering only truly righteous prayers. The Unfathomable Divine just did not want me to have a food processor. Not only that, if I'd gotten one it might have taken me the whole month just to learn how to use the dang thing. And the clincher is this: by a fluke of fate I happen to be a whiz with a kitchen knife.

How so? In 1968–69 I was a frequent extra on soap operas. The producer recognized that I had some "je ne sais quoi" (it didn't hurt that I was married to him and we needed the money), which led to a short career as the lady at the bar or in the elevator. On days when I didn't have other work, I would watch the soaps—at first just out of vanity to see my butt butterfly across the screen. Eventually, I got hooked on the stories and developed an embarrassing soap opera habit—which is how I learned to chop, because Graham Kerr's *Galloping Gourmet* came on right after *Love of Life*. I can still see his fingers on the back of that chef's knife as he rocked it up and down along a carrot or an onion, leaving a wake of perfectly even pieces. I actually went through a bunch of onions and several knuckles practicing in my own kitchen. The *Galloping Gourmet* also showed me how to sauté, braise, poach, roast, toast, bake, broil, and fry meat, fowl, and vegetables. I learned how to make a roux, a sauce, a gravy, and a meringue.

In terms of life skills, Kerr proved to be a better professor than any I had in college.

And so it was that my chef's knife—with a little help from a mandoline and Zyliss slicer—was my noneclectic Cuisinart. No, I'm not talking about a mandolin, about using the strings of a musical instrument to slice boiled eggs. The mandoline—as well as the slicer—are hand tools that allow you, with rapid strokes, to turn fruits and veggies into thin or thick slices, thin or thick sticks, or fine or coarse grated pieces.

I make such quick work of any vegetable that I could easily be hired for an infomercial. I'm so fast, in fact, that if I am not conscious of what I am doing, I can make quick work of my knuckles as well. Really, in the time it would take for you to pull out your food processor, change blades, plug it in, do the grating or slicing, wash everything, dry it, and put it away, I could be finished and cleaned up with time to spare just using my mandoline and Zyliss slicer.

Not that I am against things with power cords. My stove, fridge, and microwave were so essential I didn't even put them on the list of "tools." I chose to list the blender because I hauled it out almost every day to turn steamed stubs of this and that into creamed soups. My Foley food mill, an ingenious hand-crank device for turning stewed fruits and veggies into thick sauces, might have been sufficient, but this wasn't a back-to-basics experiment. I don't live in the woods anymore. I live in a subdivision in a house with wall-to-wall carpets.

A word about the pressure cooker. It reduces cooking time, yes, but mine, an industrial-duty one, has served me for nearly forty years for so much more: canning fruits, vegetables, and meats; cooking dried beans in twenty minutes rather than three hours; and turning wild game into delicious, tender stews. In high school we would joke about "mystery meat" on our sandwiches. A pressure cooker can turn many mystery meats—raccoon or woodchuck, anyone?—into passable dinners.

These tools plus my basic cooking skills from Mother, home economics class, and Graham Kerr were what got me through the month of cooking my 10-mile diet.

Rediscovering Cooking

What I was discovering again, in short, was cooking. Cooking as a learned skill. Cooking as how one eats every day instead of our quick grazing in restaurants and shopping in minimarts and takeout and drive-throughs. Cooking from scratch, from what's at hand. If you can't cook, your eating is totally in the hands of the food industry. Even if you cook from recipes, you still need to know the basics of cooking.

When I started the 10-mile diet, these learned skills and the can-do attitude I acquired from years of do-it-yourself-ing helped me make 150+ yummy meals.

Had I stayed in New York, though, and remained on a career and family path, I might never have learned these household arts.

Do any of us these days—with food, food, everywhere and not a drop home-cooked—really need to know how to separate eggs, caramelize onions, whip egg whites and fold them into angel food cake? Do we need to know the difference between roasting, baking, braising, sautéing, frying, and stewing—and when to use each? Perhaps not. Perhaps it's fine to rely on the deli counter or the supermarket or the purveyors of dinner in a box or microwave bag or restaurants of every class and style to make our meals while we make money to pay for it. Perhaps it's just my passion for getting down in the guts of every aspect of life, learning how things work. Perhaps I lived in the woods too long. Perhaps I drank the Kool-Aid of a post-peak world, where such competencies will distinguish those who are happy from those who are bereft. Remember the old Boy Scout motto "Be prepared"?

Making Dishes Sing

All this improvisational creativity aside, I did have one cookbook on my shelves that actually taught me the essence of transforming ingredients not just into edible food but into rich, deep, flavorful meals. Rebecca Katz, former cook for the Commonweal Cancer Help Program, where I went on my road to recovery, wrote *One Bite at a Time*, which is about putting "yum" into healthy fresh ingredients so that people who can't keep down much food might actually want to eat. As someone who couldn't even get down a smoothie during my brief foray into chemo, I know how vital that is.

From Rebecca I learned about FASS, which stands for fat, acid, salty, and sweet. Once you've put a dish together, she says, you should check the FASS balance through taste, fixing it by adding one or more of the elements. Her FASS tools looked surprisingly like my exotics—extra virgin olive oil for fat, lemons or limes for acid, and sea salt, of course, for salt. For the sweet she uses maple syrup where I use local honey.

Looking at that list I wondered if the challenge of my 10-mile diet restrictions had activated some basic body knowledge. Maybe my "exotics" are a human need, not just a Vicki obsession. It's always comforting to think that wildness has not been completely bred out of me, that if I were dropped in a remote area without a cell phone I might still last the night.

The New Natural Food

This daily reviving of my cooking chops gave the term "natural food" another new twist. Natural didn't just have to do with how the food is grown. It had to do with how I was growing spiritually through eating this 10-mile food. In week one I began to sense food as community. Through eating within my micro food shed, I was becoming part of that food shed, particularly part of a community of real gardeners and farmers.

As I chopped Tricia's snow peas, onions, garlic, and kale for my evening meal, I realized that I was not only running any old vegetables, nor even just Tricia's vegetables, through the rat-a-tat of my knife blade; I was holding all the care and attention—perhaps even love—Tricia poured into this fresh food.

In the old days—just last month—of anywhere eating, I ate what was appetizing in the moment, balancing a largely unconscious set of criteria of crunch, custom, calories, culture, and several overlapping food pyramids and pies. I got my food from the bowels of my fridge or the packed shelves in my cupboards or the cheery aisles of my supermarket or the tempting menu in a restaurant. It was all mutt food, remix food, polyglot food. None of the ingredients had "grown up" together. They met only at the moment I threw them together into a dish.

The 10-mile diet started out as simply the latest and greatest mental criteria: food miles. It was becoming something different, though. A growing sense of not just being in but *belonging to* my community brought me warm, fuzzy comfort. I felt tucked in somewhere safe and cozy, like sinking into a featherbed. Not sappy. More like a daily allotment of hugs. Family therapist Virginia Satir is quoted as saying, "We need 4 hugs a day for survival. We need 8 hugs a day for maintenance. We need 12 hugs a day for growth."[3] Local food was starting to satisfy my hug quotient.

I wondered if I was simply insensitive to the love invested in growing anywhere food. Whose were the hands that normally fed me—or the throngs if you consider even something so simple as a spaghetti sauce? Tractor drivers. Pickers. Packers. Truckers. Stockers. No, I decided, that's different. Those were hands of underpaid employees or field hands—if any hands at all. Few hands touched the cows raised in a feedlot and shuttled through the killing machine, sent as carcasses to facilities that ran the meat from many animals through the grinders to become the pearls of meat in the sauce. Hands of migrants paid less than minimum wage probably picked those onions by the ton on long days. Hands of the Immokalee workers in Florida, the biggest tomato-growing state, picked the tomatoes. They were paid a wage that barely kept them breathing—which might be considered a net good if the tomatoes were heavily sprayed with pesticides. Who grew the garlic? The cilantro?

As I stood there chopping I wondered how far back in time or far away in culture I'd have to go to be intimate with food and the hands that fed me. I chopped faster, muttering the standard fuddy-duddy froth about "What is the world coming to?" and "What's wrong with young people?" Then "What's wrong not with them but with what they've been born into?" Then "What's wrong with me, not valuing chopping, cooking, cleaning?"

My Week Two Mystical Experience

There were three different kinds of intimacy growing.

One was the deeper friendship with Tricia and the new friend-ships with Molly and John, Loren and Patty, Belinda and Koren, and other farmers. Beginning to count on one another.

A second was this coziness growing—this sense of belonging somewhere real and literally earthy.

The third intimacy was with the food itself. I was savoring my meals more, not just because they tasted better but because I was cooking from scratch and each food required attention to flavor, tex-ture, cooking time. I began to sense the perfect fit between my body and my food. Because I must eat, my body is as attuned to food sources as any teenager is to a datable other. That I don't know myself this way is a testament to the efficacy of the industrial food system. You can lose your ability to taste, smell, hunt, and cook—and still consume three thousand calories a day.

Food. How basic. To think my whole life I thought I knew what it was. *The Penguin Companion to Food* showed me how limited my vo-cabulary for "the edible" was. It has more than 2,650 entries. Edible plants numbered in the hundreds of thousands before extinctions started picking them off. Heirloom and indigenous varieties of fruits and vegetables numbered in the many thousands. A typical produce department might have thirty to fifty different fruits and vegetables for sale.

Beyond what Tricia delivered, I began wondering what else grows here that I could eat. Looking no farther than my 10-mile woods I discovered wild foods like burdock, dandelion leaves, nettles, rose hips, and several kinds of mushrooms—and there are probably many more. We can still gather clams and seaweed from the shore and pull salmon, crabs, and other fish from the waters. Every one of these foods passed the sunlight and soil and rain of our region through its cells, cells that would provide my body with vibrant nutrition.

I felt like I was becoming a tad indigenous through this 10-mile experiment. I had never before thought of the plant world as a system with me as an element of it—the planter, the gleaner, the eater, and eventually—let's be honest—the eaten. The whole system had been abstract at best, like when you read a paragraph in your science book about the hydrological cycle but then leave it to experts to make sure it works in your favor—that potable water flows from the tap. I don't even need the wisdom of my ancestors to drink.

I'd lived once before in a rural farming community where I learned to garden, hunt, forage, and preserve food. I knew a bit of the camaraderie of people who depend on the land and their hands for the food they ate.

New to me, though, was how perfectly designed I am as an animal to eat what is all around me. Talk about intimacy!

Tastes came alive. I began to appreciate my very taste buds, which are exquisitely designed to receive what the natural world has to offer—the bitter, sweet, salty, sour, and umami (savory) of it—enhanced by my nose responding to those aromas from seeds and leaves, crushed and chopped and rubbed and ground into powders. Combine taste and smell with the pleasures of crunchy and creamy and fragrant and you have a symphony of tongue delights. Food and our tongues are made for each other! There is little in life as intimate as food entering our bodies and becoming us, yet how often do we marvel at this marriage of tongue and nose and sight, at the ritual of preparing the food to enter us, at that moment when sensation leaves conscious awareness until the stomach grumbles again. How often do we see the ordinary anew?

If you have nary a mystical bone in your body, skip the next few paragraphs, but I invite the rest of you to join me standing in my yard one day in September, looking at my garden, wiggling my toes into the unmowed grass, breathing the soft air and contemplating what *The Penguin Companion to Food* and my 10-mile experience were teaching me. I felt something ripple through my body. I felt food. I was in it. I felt the animals and fungi and beneficial plants and ripening fruits, and felt not just my nose and eyes responding but my skin, which nigh on quivered in response. Eyes seemed to open in the backs of my legs and my spine and hands, in my ankles and heels and shoulder blades. I was "seeing" food in total surround. Our eyes face front. Does that lead us to pursue our desires, to lurch forward into markets and bars and new cities and books, seeking nourishment for body, mind, heart, and soul? These eyes all around me gave me a relaxed sense that I need not pursue food. Nature was not designed perversely, as if it were a game of winners and losers. It was designed so that everything—including me—fit together. We are not against one another. We are for one another. This doesn't just mean rooting (so to speak) for one another winning. It means that "just rightness" of pollen and stamen, of ruminant and grasslands. Yes, due to droughts and diseases, some people—like in the dust bowl in the United States—do not survive, but "tooth and claw" is now considered a lesser evolutionary strategy than cooperate and win.

The feeling was somewhere between creepy and ecstatic. If I live in food, I can relax. Not only do I belong to my farming community and gardeners and farmers' market, not to speak of the markets that contained food I could eat again in a few short weeks; I belong here. Here. I belong to the fertility of the soil and the exquisitely adapted plants and wildlife. Perhaps the animals in this rich coastal environment felt this way and didn't even have to label it. The bear lumbered to the water's edge in the spring as walls of fish migrated upriver to spawn. They simply feasted there the way we do at an all-you-can-eat buffet. The Haida and Tlingit knew where the berries and the camas and the mushrooms and the clam beaches were and walked around in this food, eating.

The creepy part is that when you realize how deeply you depend on another—be it a berry bush or a mate—you know your vulnerability to loss. You realize that control is ultimately an illusion. We can delay death but we have not conquered it. We can build levees but we cannot control the vehemence of storms. We can, as farmers know, plant and tend and water and watch, but we only work with nature, not command it. Especially now, as we watch the skies and wonder if the storms sweeping in again and again are harbingers of climate change or just—as we hope—El Niño or La Niña.

I've discovered over many years of trying to find love without making myself vulnerable that it doesn't work. To be touched deeply, we have to open. To open is to not know or control how things turn out. Food vulnerability is the last thing any of us wants. In fact, agriculture is our sustained human attempt to control our food supplies. Without predictability of "food income," the energy of a family or culture is necessarily focused on survival. Once those needs are met, we liberate our hands and minds for invention, for the arts, for dreams, for so much of what we identify as human. So my sense of belonging to this living web of eaters and food was awe-ful in both senses of the word. It inspired awe and it pulled back the *Wizard of Oz* curtain on my safe little life where food was guaranteed. Even when I lived in the woods on a hundred dollars a month, I never wanted for food. That hundred dollars bought a lot of rice and beans, powdered milk, and peanut butter.

That fusion with the life around me and in me could not have lasted more than half an hour. I can't consciously attend to anything much longer than that. I have been able to re-create it ever since, though, by imagining that I have eyes in my shoulder blades and the small of my back and feeling myself bathed in air and light and that buzz of vitality as every scrap of life exchanges energy with what surrounds it. We breathe out and leaves breathe in. Sunflowers turn toward the sun. Our digestive tract undulates, moving food from tongue through every stage of transforming the nourishment into us and the rest into poop—which in nature would soon be soil for more to grow. I took time now to relish that experience of life moving through life and becoming life once again.

Pigging out on Tricia's food became impossible. Not only would it dishonor the life energy she invested in growing it, it would dishonor the life energy of the food itself.

Mind you, I never want to lose control over my food supply. I never want to go a day without food unless I've chosen to fast, knowing there is food waiting for me at the end of that long hungry tunnel.

Yet I never want to lose this newly awakened intimacy with food, this transforming relationship with food. Flavors and fragrances are now triggers for awe and gratitude as well as for grabbing and gobbling.

I can't tell you what I did after this moment of awe faded. I probably went upstairs to eat.

Which brings us back to the practicalities of the 10-mile diet. From talents (how to cook) and taste (how to enhance flavors) to tools (how to slice and dice, shred and shake, blend and beat, what turned out to be a mountain of food).

By the end of the second week I was surely getting the hang of my 10-mile eating. I'd do my weekly pickups on my bike—milk at Belinda's, then cheese at Nina's, then home.

This week I decided to ride over to Tricia and Kent's just to see my food ripening in the ground and on the trees. Unlike in the past when I took as an article of faith that one doesn't just "drop in unannounced," I now felt free to visit them. We were in cahoots in a daily adventure of feeder and fed. I commented in the blog about this:

> For this month, at least, it seems that Tricia and I are engaged in an equal exchange. She wakes up in the middle of the night fearing I might starve. I do too. No, seriously, this challenge is growing her as a market gardener, and the cost is a box of veggies and a dozen eggs a week. I am examining my relationship with food—and really the food system—and all it costs is 500 words a day. Blogging for food. Would that work in a pinch if I stood by the road with a cardboard sign?

Tricia was in her processing shed, a 10-by-30-foot well-built (by Kent) structure between her yard and garden where she processes and packages her bounty for market. It's well ordered and clean, with a sink, a hose with a spray head, an industrial salad spinner the size of a washing machine tub, glassine bags, net bags, twist ties, bags, and bins.

"The tomatoes are coming in, let's look," she says. I'm excited to see what's growing—and maybe glean a few castoffs unfit for the market though perfectly nutritious and delicious.

As I said earlier, she now splits the half-acre garden—ninety raised beds in all—with Pam, and each has a 16-by-55-foot hoop house (a greenhouse made of plastic pipe and clear plastic sheeting) funded by a benefactor who regularly rewards women with courage and projects with vision on our island. Indeed, the tomatoes were in. I have never tended a tomato plant that looked half as healthy as Tricia's, which stand tall between wire supports.

I felt like some jealous and dejected housewife in a 1950s ad for laundry detergent. With furrowed brow she peers over her backyard fence at her neighbor's spanking-clean, dazzling-white T-shirts and linens flapping on the clothesline. "How does she do it?" the voice-over says. "My T-shirts have [dark music starts playing] ring around-the-collar."

That's what I thought about these plants with no brown curly leaves, no slug-gutted fruit hanging limply along the bottom, no blossom-end rot.

Then I noticed, as we walked down the row, that Tricia was tidying up like a nursemaid tending tykes for impeccable wealthy parents. She clipped off brown-edged leaves, picked up the fruit that had dropped, picked out stray weeds. In part, it's because she is simply like that with everything she cares for—including me. Careful, attentive, respectful of each leaf and fruit and person. In part too it's because this is her livelihood. I am in her workshop, on the floor of her plant . . . so to speak. She also invited me to pick as many cherry tomatoes as I wanted, which I did. We exited and she tossed the "litter" she'd collected onto the huge compost mountain along the fence.

There are many theories about how to make "the perfect compost."

There's hot compost and cold compost, there's worm bins and leaf bins, and all manner of expensive containers and secret formulas. Here Tricia and Pam are the soul of casual. They have so much plant matter to toss that it all goes into a heap. I spied a "perfectly good" bok choy plant. Take off the wilt and it would be fine. Tricia saw it and saved me the embarrassment of begging by handing it to me (it was good for two meals). I put it into my backpack along with the tomatoes.

As we walked to my bike she picked up a few slightly wormy apples from the ground, looked at me quizzically, and of course I added them to my haul, hugged her, and off I went to Belinda's for the milk.

The Raw Milk Controversy

It was my third trip up the rutted dirt driveway, onto the worn wooden porch, past the Mr.-Ugly-contest-winner pooch to get my half gallon of creamy milk from the little fridge.

Belinda happened to come out and we chatted. She's well informed, feisty, and nobody's fool. She and Koren have made a life to their liking for themselves, raising animals for milk, eggs, and slaughter.

Belinda told me about the controversies surrounding raw milk—naturally from the point of view of someone who thinks it's perfectly safe and wholesome. I am still finding it hard to believe that she and I are engaged in an illegal act. The libertarian in me balked at the government sticking its nose in this neighborly trade. I was willing to sign a release form stating that I would not hold Belinda and Koren liable, even if my gut were in an uproar due to salmonella in the milk. I trusted them and believe that people-in-community take care with one another—making wholesome potluck dishes and pies for bake sales as well as trading fresh milk. This is one of the underpinnings of buying local—you know your producers and can decide whom to trust. You don't need the government to protect you from them. True, children can't make that kind of considered decision, so one would need more caution—but not a blanket rejection.

From 1998 through 2009, the Centers for Disease Control and

Prevention received notice of ninety-three outbreaks due to consumption of raw milk, resulting in nearly two thousand illnesses, only 10 percent of which sent anyone to the hospital.[4] Of course, we'd like to have zero illnesses but two thousand in eleven years isn't an epidemic. Let's put that in perspective. How many people have eaten tainted spinach in that time? Deadly cantaloupe? How many people have sickened from E. coli in hamburger meat? We don't ban meat because it could be eaten undercooked, though we might put a warning label on it about careful handling.

Of course we all want the FDA and USDA and CDC to be vigilant so that our national daily bread—nearly four tons of it consumed every twenty-four hours—will not poison us. Even so, we must, with all that fresh food sold daily, assume that the consumer is also responsible for making informed choices and engaging in safe practices.

Raw milk, it seems, is one of those front lines in the struggle between individual liberty and government oversight. In some cases, like Medicare for all, I'm for giving the government the power and pocketbook to make us one nation, all insured, with liberty from bank-breaking medical bills and fair access to health care for all. I'm for most of the ways government functions to level the playing field, giving everyone a fair shake. I'd rather have traffic lights than traffic accidents. I'd rather have local taxes than local potholes. But in the case of what we do to our own bodies—be it smoke cigarettes or have sex or drink (booze or milk)—I favor the right to choose.

For my 10-mile month, since I'm a milk drinker until I find a compelling reason to swear off the stuff, I needed to side with Belinda both on the safety of Elsie's milk and on the insanity of it being illegal for her to provide me with my weekly milk "fix."

She told me what she'd have to do to sell her milk legally. She would get a license—it's only fifty-five dollars—but that is only the beginning of an expensive and tedious process that knocks most small producers out of the market.

"The whole milking facility," she said, "requires more stainless steel than a Microsoft exec's kitchen. It has to be completely separate from the home, including bathrooms." In addition, farmers have to keep extensive records that can be inspected at any time. They also have to conduct monthly bacterial testing (at their own expense), including for Q fever, which isn't even transmitted to humans through cow's milk. The time and expense of these requirements mean that small producers (i.e., neighbors) can't afford to fly above the radar.

If you sell milk, you must comply. And the Department of Agriculture defines selling as "offering for sale, holding for sale, preparing for sale, distributing, dispensing, delivering, supplying, trading, bartering, offering as a gift as an inducement for sale of, and advertising for sale in any media."

"This means," Belinda said, "that even if you give milk away, barter, or trade milk for other items, you must meet all of the state licensing requirements."

I asked a former dairy farmer about raw milk and she said, "All milk needs to be pasteurized to be safe. But," she said as an aside, "I drank raw milk growing up and I think that's why I've traveled the world and never gotten sick." Advocates say that the bacteria in raw milk actually make our immune systems stronger.

It was easy drinking Belinda and Koren's milk. It was rich and delicious, and the thick yellow cream made wonderful butter. It came from neighbors I had come to trust. It was not easy, though, translating my personal choice into some general social policy.

Was raw milk more like alcohol or unprotected sex—risky but basically up to the individual to regulate? Was it like "consenting adults"—a transaction between two responsible individuals that didn't of itself hurt anyone else? Or more like builders who use substandard materials, risking the lives of many unwitting people should the structure fail? Where is the line between private right and public good?

I'd never until now had to tease this apart . . . for milk, of all things! In fact, this issue showed me that I had a sketchy food ethic, if any at all.

What unexamined assumptions did I have about food? Food preferences—like a spot of milk for my morning cup of tea—are one thing. Food orthodoxies—raw milk is good for you/bad for you—are quite another. How do I develop an "internal locus of control" or "agency" (psychological terms for inner authority) in my eating? In a sea of manufactured foods, many—called functional foods—claiming health benefits, how do I become an informed chooser? Whom do I believe? How do I educate myself enough (but not obsessively) to choose well what food to make my own? Literally, to ingest so it will become me.

I certainly had a lot to chew on as I tucked into my pannier a week's worth of elixir or poison, depending on who's talking.

And chew I did on my ride home—or should I say ruminate in honor of the animal in question?

My 10-mile diet led me to a raw milk supplier. My growing appreciation for the milk and my milkers led me to grumble as I rode against the corporate control of what I am allowed to eat. As Belinda says, we have lost confidence in our capacity both as animals and as citizens to make our own choices about something so basic as food. Have we replaced personal responsibility, common sense, and traditional culture with an arm's-length legal system that makes lawsuits our main recourse and corporations more trustworthy than our neighbors? I wondered how else I might have decided I was unqualified to do something so basic as eat—and thus turned authority for my food choices over to the "experts."

I arrived home, carefully poured off the cream from my jar of milk for churning later, and set it in the door of my fridge. My mind was still churning, though. What do I really believe about eating? That my body is sturdy, able to remake itself each day from any old crap I put in it? That my body is a temple and needs to be fed the most pure and nourishing substances to spur my spiritual growth? That my body is eternally too fat and needs to be fed less, period?

Let's check out some myths together—myths that convince us that cooking and eating food grown closer to home is more expensive, less convenient, more dreary, and less secure than "food court" food or industrial food or fast food or convenience food or any other type of food that requires nothing from you but money.

Fast Food Costs Less?

It's common to defend fast food based on economics. "I can't afford local food, and certainly the poor can't afford it." But it's also pretty easy to challenge this assertion.

Yes, superficially, fast food seems to solve the challenges of people with two jobs and four mouths to feed. Especially if they haven't learned to cook from scratch—or cook much at all. It's a revolving door: the fast food industry makes it easier to fill your family's calorie (if not nourishment) needs inexpensively, so you don't exercise your cooking skills, which atrophy . . . which makes fast food ever more necessary. Not everyone wants to reverse that process in their own lives. It does take time and work, just like breaking any other habit. As I've said, affordability is one of my hardest nuts to crack (if I had nuts!). Here's how I'm doing it.

A McDonald's Quarter Pounder, on average, costs three dollars. A quarter pound of local grass-fed beef costs me $1.25. You might like it just as much—unless you miss antibiotics and stress hormones in your meat, not to mention extra fat, which may well carry pesticides, herbicides, etc. Sliced onions and tomatoes and lettuce were available on my 10-mile diet and cost pennies. Had I the time, I might have been able to make sauerkraut (salt shredded cabbage, then cover it with a weighted plate so it brines in its own juices for a week) or even pickles. What about mayo—you can make that with oil and an egg yolk. What about ketchup? You can make that with onions, tomatoes, peppers, honey, and spices. A bun would be possible with a 25-mile diet, but for the sake of our financial calculations, let's simply buy a high-end locally baked burger bun for fifty cents. Even if you give it a squirt of anywhere ketchup you are well under three dollars. You can go eat it in the car if you miss the experience.

What about a side of fries? In the drive-through a small one will set you back a buck. With my chef's knife I can turn some big Tricia or Eric potatoes into sticks, coat them in oil, sprinkle them with salt, and put them in the convection oven until they brown. Probably a buck, but you end up with the equivalent of three sides of fries.

If you want to make this faster food, you can buy ten pounds of local burger, make it into patties, and freeze them individually. You can slice a bunch of sweet Walla Walla onions (with your Zyliss slicer) and freeze them as well.

You say you don't know how to prepare them? Aah, now we're cooking with gas, so to speak. We're back at how the industrial food system has allowed us to drift away from basic human competencies.

Am I saying there is anything inherently wrong with that fast food meal? It's your choice. I am just taking away from you the argument that it's less expensive than a local food meal. It's habit, cooking deficit disorder, advertising, social pressure (especially from the kids in the backseat), and FASS that keep you going back to these ubiquitous fast food outlets. I agree, these are powerful forces to overcome, but if you are motivated to improve your diet and empower yourself and "bless the hands that feed you," you might give it a whirl. Even for one meal a week, just as a revealing little experiment.

Let's challenge those boxed foods now, shall we? Let's examine one of the many "hamburger helpers." A box with five ounces of pasta plus spices costs $2 unless you are a super coupon buyer. That's $6 a pound for pasta—plus you still have to cook it. Or you can buy pasta for just over $1 a pound; $1.50 a pound if you go whole wheat organic. You just drop it by the handful as needed in boiling salted water and fish out the finished pasta in seven to nine minutes.

For a hamburger dish that looks like the picture on the box and tastes better, sauté your burger meat, add the spices you like, make a sauce by adding some cream to the burger drippings, and voilà, you have the same meal, only 20 percent of the cost.

Same for tuna helper. Or a vegetarian pasta dish with grated cheese, olive oil, and sautéed broccoli or zucchini and onions.

Sure, pasta isn't local for most of us, but wait a decade—as local food becomes both more common and more necessary you'll have grain farmers in your region and pasta makers too (pasta is just wheat, eggs, oil, salt, and some good coaching).

Am I dissing Hamburger Helper? Not really. I'm dissing the conditions that make us believe it's in any way the best way to feed your family a nutritious meal.

A friend cooks a pot of brown rice on Sunday and uses it all week in various dishes. With a rice cooker you combine a two-to-one ratio of water to rice, add a bit of salt and oil, click it on, and wander away. You do the same with a pot on the stove, but if you walk away, come back in twenty minutes for white rice, forty minutes for brown, take it off the heat, fluff it with a fork, and let it cool.

What about a Taco Bell–like treat? Sauté your burger, shred some lettuce and dollop with a quarter cup of canned refried beans and lettuce, and you have a cheap home-cooked meal. Or you can get dried beans for a fraction of the cost of canned, cook them in a slow cooker, and mash them when they are soft. If you have a pressure cooker and know how to use it (not hard, especially if you read the manual), you can turn any kind of dried beans into dinner with half an hour of cooking after soaking them overnight.

How much are you paying a day for that fast food lunch? Three dollars? Four? Six? You can bring a sandwich to work. Or boiled eggs, apples, carrots, raisins, and almonds. You'll feel so virtuous that you'll lose weight just by hours of exercising your smugness, not to speak of how healthy that all is.

Breakfast? Forget about the drive-through. Microwave a yam. Really, it's a great breakfast. Or before you go to bed, put a handful of oatmeal plus some raisins, chopped nuts, and cinnamon in a wide-mouth thermos, pour about triple the amount of boiling water over it, tighten the lid, and you'll have warm oatmeal in the morning. Or buy bulk (not packaged!) instant oatmeal and make it in the morning. Pour on some milk and you'll have a super-healthy breakfast. How hard is it to scramble a few eggs? Grate some cheese (or crumble some goat chèvre) on them and they'll taste really rich. With toast that's

$.60 for the eggs, $.20 for the cheese, $.20 for the toast, and some pennies for the salt, oil, and butter. An Egg McMuffin costs $1.65. My version is twice the amount of food at almost half the cost. If you regularly run out of the house late for work, consider boiling some eggs on Sunday to grab as you go out the door. Add an apple and some almonds and you've got a good meal.

This is not a recipe section or a judgment about your lifestyle. As I've said, I know that in the stress of daily routines of life on the go, we develop habits in order to squeeze everything we have to do into our busy lives. I am suggesting, however, that our time-saving habits don't have to revolve around corporate foods that commercialism has convinced us to use. And I am offering these few examples of how a short apprenticeship with someone who knows how to cook can save you money and help you turn local ingredients into cheap meals. Don't have a mom or aunt or neighbor who knows how to cook and has the time to teach you? Almost everyone and his sister has access to YouTube cooking videos.

Cooking from Scratch Takes Too Much Time?

What about the time cost of these local treats? Hmmm. Let's return to the yummy, greasy McDonald's Quarter Pounder. Here's how it works out for me on a semirural island. The closest McDonald's is forty-five miles away, so let's substitute Dairy Queen—barely inside my ten miles, though for this calculation it doesn't matter. That DQ is only twenty-five minutes—round-trip—away from my home. Add waiting for your order to be ready and it's another ten minutes. Let's compare this to your local burger. How long would it take me to slice up the potatoes and put them in the convection oven, take a patty out of the freezer, thaw it slightly, fry it, slice a tomato, rip a piece of lettuce, slap it all on bread, put it on a plate, get the fries out of the oven, and sit down in my beautiful, cozy home to enjoy this nourishing meal? Less than thirty-five minutes. Oh, and add the cost of gas to the DQ. At current prices that trip would cost at least three dollars. If you live in a city, your calculation will certainly financially favor fast food—but we are questioning assumptions here, not advocating for local as the new right way.

Okay, so doing the work yourself robs a teenager or minimum-wage worker of a job, but is this the reason you eat fast food?

I want to address the time-strapped among you. Maybe you are working two jobs to pay the bills. Maybe you and your mate both work eight-hour-a-day—minimum—jobs.

In *Your Money or Your Life,* we suggest that you translate your expenses into the time it takes you to earn the money to pay the tab. We also suggest, based on feedback from thousands of people who've done the calculation, that your real hourly wage—what you keep after factoring in job-related expenses and the extra time it takes to commute—is probably a quarter of your nominal per-hour salary. There have even been some two-hundred-dollar-an-hour consultants who, when they factored in their free introductions and their Web site writing and marketing hours, found they spend ten hours for every hour of paid work.

Median household income in the United States is currently approximately three times minimum wage, averaging twenty-four dollars an hour. Let's say that ends up being a real hourly wage of six dollars.

Two basic medium pizzas in my region average ten dollars each, or twenty dollars to feed your family. Add fries, salads, and drinks and you are up to thirty dollars minimum. Five hours of work.

When you think about the cost of foods you normally buy, cooking at home starts to look very appealing—especially with those recipe apps for your smart phone and YouTube cooking shows.

You start to wonder why you slipped into that fast food, take-out food habit. You might ask, as I now ask all the time, "Who wins if I believe cooking is beyond my capacities?" "Who wins if I think I don't have time for cooking but I do have time for TV, because I deserve it after a long day?" You might follow the money and ask, "Who profits from my not knowing how to cook from real ingredients?"

Who got us assuming that fast food is better for our time and money budgets? Did we? Or were these thoughts generated by PR departments about the "scientific research" that proves that product A, with ingredient B, will make you stronger, wiser, thinner, younger, and better?

Back to fast food. Looking at that real-hourly-wage calculation and the time cost of fast food, you might wonder how fast it really is anyway. Perhaps we should call it the industrial-food-system storefront. Or simply "impulse food," since it is designed to hook you, hungry or not.

The Extra Benefits of Cooking from Scratch

Better Health

If you cook you are more likely to use fresh whole ingredients, thus sidestepping the endless worry about which additives are bad . . . and which are worse. If you invest your time in cooking food, you may find that you invest a tad more awareness in eating it. It's easier to overeat when someone you don't know cooks the food. Besides the nutrition in fresh, whole, and nontoxic foods, there are other health benefits of cooking from scratch.

What about the stress of cooking? We think take-out food takes the stress out of eating, but does it? Cooking for me is actually relaxing. It takes me out of my mind and into my body, especially hand prep like slicing and chopping. What if you considered cooking as a destressor rather than a stressor? Who would win then?

Cooking may even keep your brain sharp too. Brain research shows that learning new things keeps your brain in shape. Just as learning a language is recommended as mental calisthenics for staying brain-buffed into old age, learning the language of spices, herbs, methods, and ingredients and discerning FASS means learning to cook is literally brain food.

What if cooking from recipes is as good as crossword puzzles, known to help seniors keep their minds active? You encounter new ingredients. You have to calculate quantities if you adjust the recipe. You use your senses: When are the onions translucent? Does it have enough salt? What is al dente? Compare this to opening a microwavable packaged dinner. Which one exercises your senses and intelligence more?

I can't prove it, but the convenience of prepared food—takeout, fast food, prepackaged food—may allow us to eat more than we should simply because it seems so easy and cheap.

Greater Togetherness

For many couples, cooking dinner together is their daily dose of togetherness. Cooking with your children gives them both parent-time and a sense of usefulness, which psychologists say are two deep desires of children. Breakfast where everyone reads the backs of cereal boxes or competes for the toaster for their Pop-Tarts doesn't add a feeling of home and family security to the day. Of course, for some parents, it simply doesn't work to engage the entire family in this way. But for the parents who would like to do so, a shift is possible, and with it, support for changes in the way we eat.

The Freedom of Resourcefulness

You know by now that I have a self-sufficiency streak. Planning for old age for me includes the possibility that global systems might not continue to seamlessly, invisibly, and inexpensively bring food, energy, and whatever income I derive from investments to my door or PO box or bank. Knowing how to cook and preserve basic food is part of my long-term strategy for freedom in the event of a future in which global systems fail.

Belinda's Wisdom

This week, after stashing Belinda's milk, I went out again on my bike, whizzing down my steep hill and heading over to Nina's for my illegal goat cheese with Belinda's words reverberating in my mind.

"Eating should be a research project too. If you don't grow/know your own food, then know your farmer and his/her practices. Verify that their actions align with their intentions. It is not enough to want to provide safe food, it requires a knowledge base and follow-through. I don't know where the answers will be found, but I believe there are many answers, not just one."

Sandra, the mother of cheese-outlaw Nina, waylaid me as I lifted my bike onto its kickstand.

"Come with me. I have something for you."

Hal and Sandra's property was small. The garden lay on a north-facing slope (the worst for gardening), yet it was lush with food, animals, fodder, and medicinal plants. The goats and chickens shared a cleverly designed octagonal shed. The milking parlor had just enough room for one goat to turn a corner and put her head through the narrow V-shaped stanchion that kept her steady for milking as she bent to eat her food. (I can identify—food steadies me as well.)

From the garden we went out to their huge garage, where she pulled something from their freezer. "I want you to have this," she said, handing me a three-pound package of a goat leg.

I was left speechless—and my friends will tell you how rare that is. The remnant of my suspicious East Coast mind asked, "Why is she giving this to me?" My West Coast mind said, "Generosity isn't an agenda, Vicki. This is a gift. The right response here is to just receive it."

I did take it, feeling both the heft of the package and the lightness of wonder at generosity. She told me about the goat whose meat I held in my arms. How it was happy from day one to day last. How they raised it and loved it. How it was born to the goats they milk now.

I guess the way to this community's heart is through my stomach, I thought as I packed Nina's illegal cheese and Sandra's non-USDA-approved goat leg in my now bulging pannier and cycled home in the waning light. I felt full. These relationships and these new thoughts were becoming as nourishing as the food I unloaded on my counter.

That goat leg was too precious to improvise a dish and fail, so I went online and found a recipe for roast lamb. With reverence for my feeders and for this small creature I would be eating, I washed the leg, poked holes all around into which I put slivers of garlic, rubbed the outside with oil, a squeeze of lemon, salt, oregano, and basil, and roasted it slowly in my convection oven.

Perfect fat/acid/salty/sweet. Perfect love. Yum!

After dinner, I blogged:

Generosity itself is kept at arm's length in our everyday lives. We click PayPal buttons. We write checks between Christmas and New Year's based on well-presented literature about people far away. But here I am being invited to eat Sandra's kid (goat). How can we not be friends in the future? . . . Food is love. Every exchange is love. More love than any of us can bear if we are honest. And so I blog to digest it all—and to celebrate another part of my food system—the humans who spread the love around.

And so ended week two of my adventure.

Now It's Your Turn

Cooking

Local ingredients, cooked with love, eaten with awareness, in the company of friends—that's relational eating.

How do you feel about cooking? Comfortable? Panicked? Unimaginative? Inept? Disdainful? Ashamed? You don't have to cook to be a relational eater, but you may want to.

If you don't know how to cook, take classes from local chefs, caterers, or friends who know how to transform local produce into local yum. There are apps or Web sites where you type in ingredients and up come user-rated recipes.

Or maybe you know how to cook but you just don't for all the common reasons: time, time, and time.

Increase your home-cooking time by 10 percent. Find regional eggs and cook your breakfast. Find regional greens and steam them to go with the box of Chinese food you brought home. Take the time to grow sprouts on your windowsill and add them to your salads. Do a home-cooked meal once a week. Or make a big soup or casserole on Sunday and eat it all week.

One brilliant aid for home cooking is the pressure cooker. It saves both time and money. You can cook whole foods like beans and grains in far less time. Because all the action is hidden and under pressure, it can be unnerving the first few times you use it. You can't peek or test for doneness. Once you get the hang of it, though, it's your friend for life in getting dinner on the table fast.

Develop Your Signature Soup

I've become a soup maker as a way to use the variety of local ingredients that pour into my home at least six months a year. Knowing the textures, flavors, and cooking behavior of my fresh foods, I now have a "signature soup"—a hearty minestrone with a touch of Indian. Here are some basics I use—not recipes but approaches:

Some things to steam or boil and then puree in a blender for a creamy soup: cauliflower, leeks, summer or winter squash, potatoes, turnips, rutabagas, parsnips, carrots.

Some things to sauté and put in soup when tender but not mushy: onions, carrots, celery, garlic, green peppers, potatoes, green beans, snap peas, broccoli, mushrooms, cabbage.

If you are an omnivore—as I am—then you can use chicken (boil bones or cook pieces and use the meat too) or beef (boil knuckles and bones) bones to make your broth.

If you are either a vegavore or an omnivore, beans and grains add heft (you'll read about Georgie, Georgina, and Lauren in chapter 9— they were my 50-mile diet suppliers). You can use anywhere quinoa, lentils, amaranth, oats, baked and chopped tubers (yams, sweet potatoes, potatoes, etc.).

Bouillon (chicken, beef, or vegetable) to make the stock if you don't have fresh.

Some other juicy elements: chopped tomatoes, chopped summer squash.

Some herbs (fresh if possible) and spices: parsley, oregano, basil, thyme, marjoram, cumin (I used to think it smelled like gym socks, but now I can't cook without it), coriander, fennel, curry (careful, some are better than others), tamari, salt, and pepper. Cilantro is good in Mexican soups.

Add at the end: chopped chard, kale, mustard greens, beet greens. These will all cook as the soup slowly cools down after turning off the burner.

Mess around with these ingredients. Check for FASS—fat, acid, sweet, salt—and adjust. I'm always surprised at how a squeeze of lemon can brighten a soup. Oh, now I really sound like a chef!

Homegrown

Growing food used to be a shared endeavor on the part of the whole tribe. Just growing sprouts on your windowsill shifts you from being a food consumer to being a food producer.

Even if you spend 99.9 percent of your time otherwise occupied, your experience as a grower will put you back in the tribe.

If you don't yet garden, here are some ideas:

- Herbs in pots on your windowsill
- Tomatoes in containers on your deck
- Greens too can be grown in containers
- Window hydroponics
- Backyard garden plot
- Take gardening classes
- Volunteer at a school, community, food bank, or market garden

Try These Recipes

It turns out there was a better local alternative to zackers. Jess Dowdell shares her kale chip recipe. Kim Bailey's rich bone marrow broth is a great example of simmering from scratch. Along with the recipe, Kim shares some of her own story.

Kale Chips

So easy and fun to have around. I just take any kind of kale, but my favorite is lacinato kale, and lightly spray it with vegetable spray. I use high-heat canola oil from Spectrum. Salt and pepper the leaves and lay them in a single layer on a baking sheet. Bake at 300°F for 30 to 50 minutes, until they are crispy. Let them cool and store in an airtight dry container. You can crush them into a powder and use it as "kale salt" over many dishes for added flavor.

And here's another chip:

Root Chips

Beets, potatoes, carrots, turnips, and parsnips are all good for this technique.

Thinly slice them, about ⅛ inch thick, then toss the slices with oil, garlic, salt, pepper, and any other herb that sounds good to you. Lay them in a single layer on a baking sheet and bake at 350°F for about an hour, until they are crispy like potato chips. Let them cool and chomp away!

Kimberly Bailey of Pickles Deli says:

> I have a little deli that opened six years ago on the south end of Whidbey Island. Eating local, organic, and sustainable is very important to me. I have my own garden and utilize several farms on the island for my restaurant and home.
>
> During the months when the crops and harvests are bountiful on the island (which is quite long, April through November) I create a menu called "From Whidbey's Palette to Your Palate." This

additional menu accompanies our standard one. This gives the customers a choice to eat local meats, cheeses, and vegetables. The menu focuses on all the fresh, local, organic, sustainable ingredients this wonderful island has to offer. I have a lot of customers look at this menu and ask, "What is a dragon langerie bean?" Or, "What is spicy lamb chorizo?" And, "Oh, I didn't know you could grow or raise that here." I love explaining who the farmers are, where the food was grown or raised, and the method of farming they use. Every second you have to educate someone on what their own community has to offer, the better knowledge they have now to use and teach someone else.

I think it is important to support the hardworking farmers because they are growing/raising items that nourish our bodies—feed our souls. With rising fuel costs and a limited fuel supply it just makes sense to grow food locally so we don't deplete all of our country's natural resources.

Grass-Fed Bone Marrow Broth

Below is the Grass-Fed Bone Marrow Broth. I use Chia Farms Dexter cattle bones, Willowood Farm produce, Midnight Kitchen bay leaves, Good Faith Farm olive oil, and Whidbey Island Winery Malbec. I adapted it for my restaurant using Sally Fallon's Nourishing Traditions broth recipe.

2–4 pounds beef marrow knucklebones—with meat on them

3 pounds meaty rib or neck bones

3 onions, coarsely chopped

3 carrots, coarsely chopped

3 celery sticks, coarsely chopped

Drizzle of olive oil

4 or more quarts cold water

¼ cup apple cider vinegar

6 peppercorns

2 bay leaves

Splash of red wine

Pinch of sea salt

Preheat the oven to 350°F.

Place all the meaty bones and veggies in a roasting pan and drizzle with a little olive oil. Brown in the oven for 30 to 60 minutes, until well browned.

Meanwhile, throw all of your nonmeaty marrow bones into a stockpot, and add the water and vinegar. Let them sit while the other bones are browning.

Add the browned bones, peppercorns, and bay leaves to the pot, deglaze your roasting pan with red wine to get up all of the browned bits, then pour this liquid into the pot. Add additional water if needed to cover the bones and veggies.

Bring to a boil and remove the scum/foam that rises to the top. Reduce the heat, season with a little sea salt, cover, and simmer for at least 12 and up to 72 hours. The longer you cook the stock, the richer and more flavorful it will be. If you find there is floating fat from the marrow or oil, skim it off with a spoon or wait until after refrigeration.

When it's done simmering, strain everything—use your hands to squeeze all the goodness out.

Stick it in the refrigerator and let the fat harden on top of the pot. When hard, scrape it off and you will have a delicious bone marrow broth.

CHAPTER SIX

Week Three:
The Week of My Discontent

Okay, enough of the mysticism. While everything I just said about wiggling my toes in the grass and merging with life is true, it's also true that by week three the self-constructed fence between me and unfettered eating was making me feel as dreary and burdened as the babushka'd peasants in one of those old black-and-white Russian epics of hardship and starvation. I know it's not rational to compare my voluntary situation to famine, but that's how it felt to me.

I was finally getting into a groove. Days went by. I blogged. I cooked. By week three I had the hang of a new, preferred 10-mile daily fare. For breakfast I ate a frittata. I'd sauté some thinly sliced onions and potatoes in olive oil, and then add julienned zucchini or chopped fresh kale from my garden, some basil, and a crushed sun-dried tomato from Tricia's prior season. I'd scramble one or two of Tricia's eggs, stir in the sautéed vegetables plus salt, and return the mixture to my well-seasoned cast-iron pan. It cooked on low heat, covered, until the edges were done and starting to brown. Then the trick is to cover the pan with a plate, flip it quickly, and return the frittata—uncooked side down—to the pan to finish. Add tea from China, milk from Koren and Belinda, and honey from Island Apiaries, and I truly had enough.

Lunch was usually a salad because Tricia supplied me amply with cucumbers, tomatoes, mixed greens, carrots, apples, basil, and sometimes even a pepper. Dressing of lemon juice, oil, and salt. Goat cheese on top.

Snacks were often big flat Italian beans from my garden, steamed and coated with oil and salt.

Dinner would be some creation utilizing frozen local meat and fresh Tricia produce. Liver and onions. Burger and oven fries. Stir-fried vegetables. Sliced tongue. Braised greens with onions and garlic. Don't I sound like quite the cook?

As long as I stayed home, in my ten miles, in my now familiar cycles of eating and cycling to gather food, I was fine.

But I was also trapped. I'm used to mobility. I'm used to going where whim, will, or necessity sends me, confident that my destination will also be filled with mountains of food. My blissy little ten-mile loop was beginning to feel more like a chain getting yanked.

In week three, for example, I wanted to attend a regional gathering of Transition Town groups. It was in Bellingham, a mere one hundred miles north. To survive for fifteen hours out of my teensy-weensy microbioregion I was going to have to schlep a day's worth of food along with me.

I packed a Conestoga wagon load of salad, bags of steamed green beans and steamed kale, a pint of milk, the entire bottle of honey (decanting was too much trouble at five A.M.), several baked potatoes and boiled eggs, carrots, and an apple.

All the while I packed the food I felt something between self-pity and irony. By choice I was sending myself back a century in time or off to a less-developed country. I couldn't moan, "Why me, oh Lord," because it was evident that I had brought this on myself.

I was brought up to think about those less fortunate, so my thoughts then turned to people I've known who have food sensitivities and must pack this way all the time. Allergies to wheat, dairy, gluten, chicken, oats, nitrites, peanuts, tree nuts in general, beef, eggs, shellfish, seafood, and soy are increasingly common. I once stumbled on a few people living in a tent colony in the desert who had just about every sensitivity in the book. They were like people quarantined—struck with the plague—except they had to keep us out to survive. Any whiff of perfume could send their bodies into a complete tizzy, and soap, detergent, deodorant, baby powder, shampoo, conditioner, face cream, salves, and toothpaste all stink to them. There are now thirteen thousand name-brand perfumes alone. I was quarantined—voluntarily—only to a ten-mile radius for a month. You are not suffering! I scolded myself. You are being slightly inconvenienced. Stop whining.

Wine. I'd love a sip of wine, yet at that time none was purely local.

See. I could say "Get my goat" or "Don't cry over spilled milk" or "That sounds fishy," and my nose would start sniffing the air, my tail would rise, and I'd be ready to hunt again.

Yet this sense of deprivation was chosen and time-limited—and still something of a lark. The problems of the ill and underprivileged endure for weeks, months, and even lifetimes. On October 1 I could release my chosen constraints. But those with fewer resources often live in what are now called food deserts, city neighborhoods where the poverty rate is 20 percent or higher and the nearest healthy, affordable food is a mile or more away.[1] Even more reason for me to refrain from whining.

Still I kept on. My lovely cup of morning tea was now not ginger and not orange juice and not a banana smoothie. I sipped it as I waited for my ride to Bellingham, surrounded by what now seemed a steamer trunk full of food, and sniveled more.

I looked for an apt analogy for how I was feeling and could find none better than the very Russian peasants I mentioned earlier. My mother and I journeyed to Russia back in the days when it was still the USSR—back when travel was all but banned and the few tourists allowed to enter had to travel via Aeroflot planes (think of flying Model T Fords) and stay in former czarist palaces converted to Supreme Soviet–approved fleabag hotels with only cold running water and room keys made for dungeons. She was attending—of all things—a psychological meeting in Moscow. Back then we thought that Russians used mind control to quell the toiling masses. They made people psychologically ill, not well, or so the stereotype went. I was curious to travel behind the Iron Curtain and was along for the ride.

We'd flown from Latvia to St. Petersburg on an international airline, but the St. Petersburg to Moscow flight was entirely Russian and entirely different. Clutching our passports as if they were parachutes, we boarded our Aeroflot plane for our flight. Along with us—I kid you not—came a family carrying their chickens in a cage. Bringing fresh food for the journey meant bringing it live for slaughter at their destination.

I flashed back to all those third-class train rides I'd taken the year before when I studied in Spain. There too lumpy older women, black scarves tied around their doughy faces, toted large baskets of food on their trips. Later I'd see the same sight in India, China, and Southeast Asia. The local passengers knew not to assume there would be food when the train stopped in the dead of night because a cow was on the tracks or something broke and they had to wait for another train to pick them up. In two days.

Or perhaps they were taking a family member to the hospital, where they would need to cook for the patient—probably a big improvement over the institutional hospital food we get here.

Surviving the Day

My friends arrived to pick me up for our carpool to Bellingham. Without Sherpas I had to lug my bags down my front stairs to their car, feeling dowdier by the minute. Their cheerfulness snapped me out of my mood. I refocused on how far less common food scarcity is in this country; we are actually so awash in food that we throw out one third to one half of it somewhere between the field and the Dumpster. How lucky we are to be confident that wherever we go, food will be there to greet us.

We arrived two hours later. Sixty bright, creative people from Transition groups in the region eagerly swapped stories, insights, and challenges for a rich day of conversation. Everyone but me feasted at the snack and lunch tables. I, the self-excluded, nibbled through my stores, gauging hour by hour whether my food would last. By dinner I had three green beans, two carrots, and an apple left. The gnawing hunger in my gut hammered at my virtuous mind. You don't have to starve, I said to myself. You don't have to be such a purist. The exception proves the rule—let dinner be your exception. This is just an experiment, not an assignment from on high.

And on and on. I was afraid, though, to fall off the local food wagon. I might not have the will to get back on. My word seemed my only protection from lapsing.

As this little skirmish went on in my mind, Chris Wolfe of Transition Whatcom County took the microphone to announce that dinner was ready. As she described every ingredient and the local farmer who grew it, my resolve began to waver. She had personally looked in the eye of almost every producer for the fare she offered—greens, beets, soups, granola, apples, eggs, cornbread, berries, even lentils. What wasn't a direct buy was bought from local organic grocers.

The food was as local as she could get, and given that she was feeding sixty people three meals that day and had never before fed more than nine people at one meal, the love in that meal—love like a fierce commitment to nourish the tribe—was immense.

"I haven't slept much the last few days," she said. "Oh, and I've prayed I wouldn't make any of you sick." She was as radiant as if she'd just run a marathon and this was her finish line. By eating, the group would be partaking of her victory.

I began to feel more like a sourpuss than a lover of the hands that feed me.

Then she said, "There's plenty of food. Even if you didn't sign up for a meal, you're welcome to eat. Everyone should have enough to eat. Be my guest."

That did it. In this space of love and generosity my rigid loyalty to my 10-mile food seemed petty rather than noble. To turn down food is one thing. To turn down love is another. I caved. My stomach did a little victory dance as I loaded up on spinach salad and lentil soup and sat with my new friends.

As we chatted over the meal I wondered whether in fact this food was more 10-mile food to me than what I'd hauled from my micro food shed a hundred miles south. Is 10-mile eating ultimately honoring the locale you are in, rather than a peevish insistence that only food from your patch of earth is local? Maybe our 10-mile circle moves with us as we move our bodies. Maybe the love shining in Chris's eyes was more to the point than loyalty to my micro-foodshed.

Going Local, Wherever You Are

I was back in the circle of community, returned from the land of feeling deprived and excluded, warmed by companionship, fed. The lessons, however, would never leave me.

The first lesson is that love trumps pride—or can when we're faced with big challenges and community is crucial to surviving. Then we discover what's important and who are "our people."

The second lesson is what Mark Twain advised: "Moderation in all things, including moderation." It's hard—but doable—to eat locally wherever you are. In Bellingham, that would be Whatcom County. On Whidbey it's Island County. Ultimately, though, local isn't just a ten-mile spotlight that travels with me, showing me what I can eat. Local means being in relationship with the hands that feed me, whether it's a two-hour walk from home or a two-hour drive or a two-hour flight. In addition to being about the environment, about sustainable local communities, and about healthful foods, it's about nourishing closeness.

Distance, then, isn't the new, improved measure of food correctness. Fear of the post-peak-oil future, with collapsed food-supply chains and cars bumping along potholed roads burning the last drops of fossil fuel, is too small and paranoid a motivation. Community, though, is a delicious reward for local eating, whether or not we get our civilizational comeuppance.

I prefer blessed-if-you-do, blessed-if-you-don't scenarios. I choose to try new behaviors that will certainly stand me in good stead should the global supply chain break down but will also make my life richer and happier even if the whole industrial enterprise self-corrects and survives for centuries to come.

The Transition movement partakes of this same blessed-if-you-do, blessed-if-you-don't attitude. Transitioners are passionately engaged in resilience (diversifying local economies), resourcefulness (creatively using and repurposing what is already at hand to solve problems), and relocalization (reducing dependencies on long supply chains for our food, water, energy, tools, and stuff of daily life). These three together—resilience, resourcefulness, and relocalization—are the key to thriving in these uncertain times.

Resilient systems are diverse, networked rather than hierarchical, sharing rather than hoarding, collaborative rather than competitive, communicative rather than secretive. They flourish by increasing options and strategies for the system as a whole. Resilient people are resourceful—able to meet their needs in a wide variety of ways.

Relocalization is the process of communities becoming resilient and people becoming resourceful—so that we have more and more local options for meeting more of our needs. This is the inspiration and aspiration of Transition Towns. There are critiques of these multiplying efforts (approaching a thousand communities worldwide). They are accused of being

- Pie in the sky: at best another marginal movement, this generation's "back to the land."
- Xenophobic: abandoning the world's problems, building a local fortress, and pulling up the drawbridge.
- Regressive: human destiny lies in our mastery of life, not in our adapting to limits.
- Unnecessary: the global economy will—as it always has—wobble and right itself. Some individuals may suffer along the way, but the arc of history bends toward material progress.

Most of the time, this nay-saying rolls off my back. If resilience, resourcefulness, and relocalization prove to simply be lifestyle choices and not lifeboats, so what? The emotional, spiritual, and relational benefits far outweigh the "rewards" of consumerism. Will it turn the tide or turn out to be one more good (alternative) college try? So what, if it is fulfilling, empowering, and fun for those who do it?

October Surprise: It's Not Over!

There was one unexpected result of that Bellingham experience. Someone there said to me in a "gotcha" way, "All well and good to do this experiment in September. Try doing it in January." Smirk, smirk. What I wanted to say was, "You try doing this in September and then get back to me." But I didn't. I just started to calculate how I would do it in January. I could tinker with the "it" a bit, expanding the radius and including more exotics. I could also do "it" in February so "it" didn't feel like New Year's penance for the wanton gluttony of the holidays. Plus February has three fewer days than January.

What if local meant a circle that includes Whidbey and Bellingham, includes Island, Skagit, Whatcom, Snohomish, King, and Jefferson counties—which together might be a viable, diverse, resilient food system for all who live in their bosom.

For today, it was enough to expand the definition of 10-mile eating to include eating locally wherever I found myself. But from February, what might I learn?

As I dozed in the car on the way home from Bellingham, tummy full, friends packed around me like sardines, the phrase "50 percent within 50 miles in February" floated to the surface. That had a ring to it. I'll do it, I said to myself. I was back in my sustainability-as-an-extreme-sport mind. But I was also nervous, as I often am when I say yes to what seems impossible but worthy. Visions of hours at the stove turning withered potatoes into paltry gruel pecked at my mind like a chicken. Indeed, I did feel chicken. But I knew I would do it.

How Much Is That Chicken in the Freezer—Tra-La?

Speaking of poultry . . . my next challenge was the five-dollars-a-pound chicken. Before this experiment began I was a chicken-a-week gal, expecting to pay no more that five to eight dollars for a bird. Now, making every effort to fulfill my promise to eat the majority of my food from Tricia's bounty, I was faced with paying for a pound what I might pay for an entire bird.

When Tricia said her neighbor Tobey raised chickens and would possibly sell a few from her freezer, I did not calculate cost. I didn't even think I had to. How much could a chicken cost, anyway?

I went over to Tobey's in a fine mood, sort of expecting that same moving experience of neighborliness I had had with Sandra. But that was not to be. Not that Tobey was anything but generous and cheerful. After all, he had a limited supply and was willing to share. It was the sticker shock when the bill came that turned that feeling of neighborliness into the reality of commerce.

Twenty-five dollars for a chicken??!! I'd never even paid that for a Thanksgiving turkey. My brain went into overdrive. I considered putting on my Shirley Temple adorable persona and cajoling that chicken out of her hands—just because I am so cute. On the other hand, Frugal Girl wanted to bargain. My starving inner Tiny Tim wanted to steal it for dinner. My omnivore just wanted that chicken—whatever the price! The inner debate raged on, but I knew that none of these characters really understood what it took Tobey to raise that chicken.

When we want to say something costs a significant amount we say, "And that's not chicken feed," as if feeding chickens were cheap. As I learned, it is not cheap at all. Let's do the math.

I checked my local friend's calculations against the chatter on the chicken forums on the Web. There seemed a consensus that factoring in . . .

- the cost of chicks,
- the cost (and quality) of feed,
- and the cost of your local electricity,

. . . the producer puts out $2 a pound in expenses to raise a chicken. Was Tobey ripping me off, then, by charging $5? No, because you have to also factor in the cost of labor.

Let's say you raise 25 chickens—how many hours a day are you tending and feeding them? One farmer in my region estimated about 20 hours of labor total for 75 chickens. Man, how does she feed, water, slaughter, pluck, gut, and pack a chicken in 16 minutes? Reading further, I saw how—she doesn't factor in the labor of her daughter and girlfriends on slaughter day. Dollars to doughnuts, as they say, she sent her daughter out to feed and water the chicks as well. And what about the time driving to the feed store and back for chicks and feed? And what about her time in the chicken chatrooms on the Internet?

I'm going to say that an honest assessment would be an hour of labor per chicken. Let's pay everyone a low wage, about $10 per hour.

For 25 chicks, the labor cost would be $250, or another $10 per five-pound chicken. Now we're up to $4 a pound.

Shall we include the cost of building and fencing a chicken house, the cost of water, or the cost of losing a chicken or two to animals or disease? Add in even a homemade chicken plucker, plus a small fraction of the taxes and insurance on your home (unless you also live in the coop), and you could say $5 a pound is easily the real cost of raising one five-pound bird.

Could I really look Tobey in the eye and say that she, with a family, should earn $10 an hour and never be able to take her brood—so to speak—out to dinner and a movie?

At the same time, Frugal Girl whined, why should I pay $25 a chicken when I can get them on sale at the Star Store for $1.49 a pound, or $7.50 a chicken? Is it my job to subsidize my local growers just because the U.S. government doesn't?

Now let's look at how the industrial producers can sell their chickens for so much less. Economies of scale (many more chickens in much less space per bird) and mechanization are key factors. For instance, the time the grower must spend on an individual bird from hatched to processed and ready for shipping is probably minutes, not hours. The big producers use biotechnology to grow bigger, meatier birds, even as confined as they are. They hatch their own chicks, saving more money. And there is labor; their workers might be getting only minimum wage, which is often quite low in Big Chicken states.

Research at Tufts University reveals one more factor—and a big one. Feed for industrial-scale chicken production is sold to the producers at below cost—thanks to government price supports and subsidies. Because my tax dollars are subsidizing the big guys but not the little guys, consider the price disparity to be due, in part, to how my government tilts the playing field toward the factories rather than the farms.

Weighing all this—the data, not the chickens—I asked myself this question: What other assumptions, habits, entitlements, misinformation, and unconsciousness made me gasp at the cost of Tobey's chicken?

Mark Bittman's Itty-Bitty Bits of Meat Diet

One big assumption to go on the chopping block—so to speak—was the amount of meat I needed per day.

During my 10-mile month I entertained myself while prepping food by watching TED talks. These are twelve- to twenty-minute presentations at TED (Technology, Entertainment, Design) hip-to-the-max conferences. The best, most interesting minds of our generation are given tight parameters about how to do a TED talk and then given a big live audience, a big PowerPoint screen, and big Internet exposure to present—briefly—their big ideas. There I found Mark Bittman, celebrity chef, cookbook writer, and columnist for the *New York Times*. He's big on a diet of vegetables, grains, fruits, and itty-bitty bits of meat. In fact, he recommends we eat only half a pound of meat a week! Folks, that's what I eat a day. This was not a welcome opinion, but I chose to keep my trap shut and mind open.

To Meat or Not to Meat?

As with so many other diet recommendations, the experts don't agree about meat.

- Vegans eat no animals or animal products.
- Vegetarians eat no animals, though they eat dairy and eggs.
- Fisho-chicko vegetarians eat Bittman-bitty amounts of animal protein.
- Omnivores eat what they like—which could range from organic grass-fed beef to a McDonald's burger.
- Paleo dieters believe in meat.
- Weston Price advocates are practically religious in their belief that animal flesh and fat has not only been given a bad rep, it's an essential part of a healthy diet. They eat butter and well-marbled (grass-fed) steak. They boil bones (especially bovine knuckles) to make nourishing broths. They believe organ meats from wild animals are especially healthy food.

I've wavered in my choices, wanting to be "good" but also wanting to eat "good"—as in yummy—meat.

As I mentioned, John Robbins's first book, *Diet for a New America,* got me off eating beef, unable to stomach the facts about animal cruelty.

When I read *Eat Right for Your Type* by Peter J. D'Adamo, I went back to beef as an essential part of a type O diet. In fact, this cured a tropical affliction I'd picked up in the jungles of Thailand.

By the time I watched Colin Campbell's *Forks Over Knives,* about the health benefits of a vegan diet, I'd already yo-yoed enough. I didn't want to do anything about it—even if it was right.

When I read the environmental argument: that ten pounds of grain are needed to raise one pound of meat—and we can eat grain—my habit and heritage fought back. Meat for protein for me wasn't just a choice. It was an article of faith.

I grew up with a food pyramid that had meat at the broad base. My mother served meat with every meal. As I learned to cook, I was told a plate must be balanced: starch, vegetable, meat. By the time I was an adult I firmly believed that animal protein was both the basis of a good diet and the pinnacle of good eating.

Now Bittman's ideas were biting me. Would I actually be healthier if I ate half the meat? Because I really like meat in all its hearty, fatty glory.

Since I was, thanks to the 10-mile diet, in myth-busting mode, I asked, Who wins if I believe I must eat three pounds of meat a week? I imagined swallowing a commercially grown chicken a week and wondered, Had I swallowed the industrial food story hook, line, and sinker? Was Bittman's argument the duh-uh truth?

My faith in meat protein teetering, I considered Bittman's claim again. Meat in moderation rather than the meal. Enjoy animal protein this way, or by eating milk, cheese, and eggs in all the many ways we do. That attitude made sense. I decided to keep it for now and see if I wanted to keep it for good.

Why Should Chicken Be Cheaper Than Beef?

From this perspective, five dollars a pound for chicken was Goldilocks's Golden Mean—not too much, not too little, but just right—at least for my budget. If I ate less meat per meal, I could now survive on two chickens a month rather than four, so that five-dollars-a-pound chicken starts to compete with the "free-range" chicken that's usually about two dollars a pound at the grocery store. (Especially knowing that *free range* might mean only that the chickens simply have a chance, like any prisoner, to walk around a small fenced yard every day, not that they're pecking at grubs in lush fields of grass.) Of course a really free-range organic bird, like the ones from Organic Prairie, the meat-producing arm of the Organic Valley Dairy Cooperative, sells for about five dollars a pound, so if you want quality meat from happy(er) birds, that does seem to be the price you'll pay. But if I started eating half as much chicken my food budget would stay the same. Frugal Girl was happy again. She'd halved the cost by halving the portion.

Having worked through all this, the next thing I realized was that if you compare the price of local chicken to the price of local beef you'll wonder what the fuss is about. Lean ground Long Family burger was five dollars a pound, just a little more than ultralean industrial beef at the supermarket. Why do we assume chicken is worth less than beef? The size of the brain? If so, why do we accept that salmon in the supermarket is minimally seven dollars a pound? To say something is cheap or expensive, you have to ask: compared to what?

So five-dollars-a-pound chicken it was, and here's the final consideration about why it is worth it. Taste. I'll tell you in chapter 7 about how that local chicken tasted. After reading my description you might well decide to raise chickens in your backyard no matter what the cost!

Where's the Wheat?

By week three I would have paid five dollars a pound for anything made of wheat if I could have gotten my hands on it. As you know, my hunt for crunch bordered on insanity. Sadly, no wheat grew within range. Or so I thought until a visit with Eric and Britt after another milk pickup. When I bemoaned for the umpteenth time my lack of crackers, Eric said, "I planted five rows of wheat as an experiment, but after the rain it molded and I'm not going to use it." Within minutes a deal was struck.

Soon I stood in that patch of mildewing wheat trying to figure out how to harvest it. I had no scythe. I had no whirling-engine mower. So I borrowed some scissors and clipped the heads off one row, filling a big shopping bag.

Once home I wondered, "Now what do I do?" I remembered the women in Thailand working a food pedal thresher. I remembered lovely *National Geographic* photos of African women winnowing grain by tossing it repeatedly in big round baskets, letting the wind take away the chaff. I remembered the big millstone I'd seen that had been turned by donkeys tempted ever forward by bags of feed just out of reach. Threshing. Winnowing. Grinding. How hard could that be?

I was determined not to lay my head down without downing at least one homemade cracker. Somehow. I am nothing if not resourceful.

To thresh the wheat I put it in a wide-mouth jar and plunged my hand mixer down into it, breaking up the wheat heads and spinning off some of the chaff. I dumped the results into a colander and broke it up more by grinding it into the colander holes with a rubber ball. Okay, I had some wheat berries and lots of chaff. Now what?

Aha! The hair dryer! I took the colander outside, plugged my hair dryer into an outlet by the door, straining the cord so I could get as far away as possible. Pointing the dryer away from the house, I shot a few blasts of air that sent the chaff swirling up, up, and back in my face as a breeze blew by. My hair and clothes were dotted with chaff, but the berries stayed mostly in the colander. A few more chilly blasts and I had a cup of wheat for my hoped-for royal bit of bread.

To turn my berries into flour, I got out my handy-dandy coffee grinder, filled it with grain, whirred it until the rattling stopped, and indeed, when I lifted the lid there was something in there that looked like flour. And all it took was a jar, a hand mixer, a colander, a rubber ball, a hair dryer, and a coffee grinder to get it. Oh, and some fossil fuel.

Of course there is no baking soda in my ten miles, much less baking powder. But salt and oil are already on my exotics list, so I mixed flour, honey, salt, water, and oil, and something came out of the pan that looked like the ancient bread the Hebrews took with them when they fled Egypt.

But I'd done it! My resourcefulness had gotten me four little pancakes with just ninety minutes of work. I slathered them (okay, dotted them) with my hand-churned butter and every bite was heaven. All ten of them.

That ironic witness who floats around amused by the antics of my daily life laughed as she watched me do my little science experiment using household gadgets. My angelic witness, though, was deeply humbled. As I thought about those women in Thailand and Africa, about those donkeys plodding in circles, I thanked my lucky stars for how far my life was from such hard, repetitive, endlessly time-consuming tasks.

The next night I shared my cracker semivictory with a friend who runs a poverty-law agency concerned with, among other issues, immigration policy. We talked about the lives of the migrant farmworkers he serves. Up at four A.M., bused to the fields, bused back at nine P.M., sleep, and start all over again. They earn about six thousand dollars a year. Less than five dollars an hour. So that I can chow down the berries and tomatoes and beans they pick in minutes? To deal with my stress? I'm forcibly reminded that I need to be more mindful of what I eat when so many people have worked for so little money to bring it to me. These are also the hands that feed me.

Kvetch, Kvetch, Kvetch

For those of you who don't know Yiddish, that means "Bitch, bitch, bitch."

If I thought that confronting my preferences was hard, confronting my privilege in this way was even harder. I was learning firsthand why "local" is practiced by only a few crazies. My next comeuppance came on my weekly bicycle milk pickup. Belinda came out the door to chat. I think she regarded me with a combination of amusement, pity, and respect.

"How's it going?" she asked, and she grinned when I admitted, "It's tough."

"You bet it's tough," she said, knowing full well that local eating isn't a sport, isn't for sissies, and isn't sincerely practiced by anyone but farmers, a few diehard eaters, and a whole bunch of free-range animals chewing local grass. She said she'd send me a link to an article on *Grist* (an online environmental news service) that would blow my mind.

She was right, and I'm excerpting it below—with permission—to give you the pleasure of that experience. It mirrors what Belinda said and I was starting to understand firsthand: that living our food values is a ball buster, a term I use because the article's author, Rebecca

Thistlewaite, does. The piece is called "So You Say You Want a Food Revolution," and it's a real call to useful action. Keep in mind that the term *farmer* used by Thistlewaite below refers to farmers of relatively small and local farms, *not* to giant industrial farms.

From your farmer—This article might challenge you, open your eyes a little more, or possibly offend a few, but the only way to make the food system better is to understand it more. Some of my most beloved clients sometimes comment about items being too expensive but I am going to answer that with a question, how many farmers do you know that live in sprawling homes and drive expensive cars? We've gotten so far away from understanding what it takes (physically and financially) to produce food that when you see it first hand it is quite surprising.

You watched Food, Inc. with your mouth aghast. You own a few cookbooks.

You manage to get to a farmer's market about once a month, but the rest of the time your eggs and meat come from Costco, Trader Joe's, and maybe Whole Paycheck now and again.

Guess what? You are NOT changing the food system. Not even close.

You're no better or different than the average American. You pat yourself on the back, you brag about your lunch on Twitter, you pity your Midwestern relatives eating their chicken-fried steak and ambrosia salad, but you secretly loathe your grocery store bill— which consumes only 8 percent of your income while your car devours 30 percent. Your bananas and coffee may be Fair Trade, but everything else is Far From It. The dozen eggs you splurge on once a month may be from local, outdoor-roaming birds, but all the other eggs you eat come from a giant egg conglomerate in either Petaluma, Calif., or Pennsylvania.

So. Want to make a difference?

Here's what a sustainable food system actually needs you to do, in no particular order:

Educate yourself:

- Learn why farmers and ranchers who don't earn enough to cover their costs are not sustainable and that something has to suffer as a result, whether it be quality, animal welfare, land stewardship, wages, health care, mental & physical health, or family life.
- Understand why sustainable food should actually cost 50 to 100 percent more than industrial, conventional food. Figure out how to buy food more directly from farmers and ranchers, if you want to avoid some of the transportation/distribution/retail markup costs.
- Understand that if you want to see working conditions and wages come up for farming and food processing workers, that you will have to pay more for food. Be OK with that.
- Learn about the Farm Bill and plan to write a letter/make a phone call when it comes up for re-authorization.

Chill out:

- Don't expect a farmer to have year-round availability and selection. Alter your diet to match the seasonal harvests in your area. Get used to not eating tomatoes until at least July, apples in late August to December, citrus in winter, greens in spring. Don't complain.
- Realize that even animal products are seasonal because animals have biological cycles. Know that chickens produce much less eggs in winter when days are shorter and even come to a complete stop when they are replacing their feathers (molting). Consequently you may have to eat less eggs and pay more for them during that time. Don't complain.
- Don't expect the farmer/rancher to sacrifice the health and welfare of the animal for your particular fad diet du jour (no corn, no soy, no wheat, no grains, no antibiotics ever, even if the animal will die, no irrigation, no hybrid breeds, no castrating, no vaccines . . . what is it this week?).
- Don't call a farmer a week before you're having a pig roast to ask

for a dressed-out pig, delivered fresh to you, for under $300. We are not magicians, just farmers.

Get your hands dirty:

- Sweat on a farm sometime.
- Participate in the death of an animal that you consume.
- If you own land that's not being farmed, tell some farmers about it. If you rent land to farmers, offer a fair rental price or fair lease (long-term is better), and then stay out of the way and don't meddle or hinder the farmers. They are not your pet farmers nor your landscapers.
- Throw your consumer dollar behind a couple beginning farmers or lower-income farmers. Be concerned about how landless, lower-income producers are going to compete with the increasing numbers of wealthy landowners getting into farming as a hobby.

Help your local farmers do their job:

- Consider making a low-interest loan, grant, or pre-payment to a farmer to help her cover her operating expenses. Stick with that farmer for the long haul, as long as he continues to supply quality product and can stay in business.
- Don't complain about prices. If price is an issue for you on something, ask the farmer nicely if he has any less expensive cuts (or cosmetically challenged "seconds"), bulk discounts, or volunteer opportunities. But don't ask the farmer to earn less money for his hard work.
- Don't compare prices between farmers who are trying to do this for a living and those that do it only as a hobby (and don't have to make a living from what they produce and sell).
- Share in a farmer's risk by putting up some money and faith up front via a Community Supported Agriculture share. And then suck it up when you don't get to eat something that you paid for because there was a crop failure or an animal illness.
- Buy local when available, but also make a point of supporting

certified Fair Trade, Organic products when buying something grown in tropical countries.

- Buy organic not just for your health, but for the health of the land, waterways, wildlife, and the workers in those fields.
- Pay for your values. If it hurts, don't have fewer values, just eat less food (sorry, but most Americans could stand to do a bit of this).

I admit, this is a lot to digest.

What I am saying is that we can't be casual about the food system we want to see. If more people don't show some commitment, and take part in some of the hard work that farmers, ranchers, and farm workers do on a daily basis, then we cannot build a sustainable food system.

You don't have to be a passive consumer. You are part of this system, too. Don't just eat, do something more!

I winced all the way through the article. I could see what it might take to really eat where my food and I are planted—and I was barely on the same planet. Whether for values or taste or ethics or belonging or ecstatic fusion with the natural world, if I wanted to be a local eater I'd need to get more than my mouth involved. If I wanted to live my values when it comes to food, I would have to do so much more. Double that if I wanted to challenge the whole dang system.

I did not—absolutely not—want to rise to that occasion. I had a life to live, a choir to sing in, a comedy troupe to rehearse with, a dance class to attend, teleclasses to teach, a house, friends, and, oh, did I mention a necessary daily full night's sleep? I was done with biting off more than I could chew, so to speak. I wanted to stay healthy and sane. I did not want to go, ahem, whole hog.

Vicki's To-Dos to Support My Farmers

I had already begun a running to-do list for supporting my local food system, should I ever want to hear the word *local* again once the experiment was over. It included the following:

1. Get farmland into the hands of young dedicated farmers like Eric—or at least get them reliable, affordable, and long-term secure access to farmland that they can invest themselves in and reap the rewards from for years to come.

2. Get the laws changed so that neighbors can sell not only their farm produce but their milk and meat, jams and jellies, canned dilly beans, and such freely to their local neighbors. Let those green libertarians among us take responsibility for the safety of our food. Don't so regulate and bureaucratize the lives of small-scale farmers that they can't legally sell to willing buyers out their back doors and in their farm stands. Yes, regulate the industrial system. Protect supermarket shoppers who want to think only about what's for dinner, not where it came from. Regulate the impersonal big guys to assure a generally safe food supply for all of us, but make "scale-appropriate" regulations for the little local guys.

Rebecca's article confirmed that if I wanted to make systemic—not just personal—change, I was already on the right track with those two points. Now I could add a few more.

3. Do something about the cost difference between local food and industrial food. At that time, I had no idea what to do, but I knew the gap between Tyson's and Tobey's chickens needed to narrow if local were to have a fighting chance in the marketplace.

4. Inform myself—and others. Stop leaving issues related to food to John Robbins and Frances Moore Lappé and Wendell Berry, to name just a few of the brilliant minds of sustainable eating and farming. Get up off your consumerism laurels and learn enough to really help.

5. Do that 50 percent within fifty miles in February. Rise at least to the challenge of a local winter diet.

We all choose how the food system grows through every choice we make—what to eat, where to shop, what to pay, who to vote for, and probably far more than I could at that moment imagine. Everything and everyone is, ultimately, part of the food system. We all eat.

The Industrial Food System Strikes Back (in My Mind)

This one-month experiment in eating hyperlocally was causing me to experience mission creep in the third week. It was threatening to occupy my life, reawaken that change maker who'd settled down as I settled in here in Langley. My better angels, of course, liked the drift of this line of thinking. My inner rabble, however, was not pleased.

We—me and the rabble—are industrial eaters to the core. I like the convenience, variety, and ubiquity of impersonal supermarket pretty-packaged food. A lot. I know it's a stage set. I know the stocked shelves of stores would empty in three days should the ferries stop running and the bridge tumble into Deception Pass. I know that more than a third of still-good food from grocery stores and restaurants is thrown away, and that food banks, freegans, and farmers with pigs to feed capture only a tiny fraction of that waste. I know that animals lead horrible lives in Concentrated Animal Feeding Operations (CAFOs). I know subsidies tilt the playing field so that my now dear small farmers struggle to make even a paltry living. I know 15 percent of Americans go hungry. I know I'm privileged beyond what I can even imagine. I know that!

I'm not talking about my conscience here. I'm talking about my deep desire to be *unconscious*, to listen only to whim, frugality, habit, preference, my body's cravings, and my mouth's unending demand for taste, volume, salt, grease, sweet. Unless you are already a food saint, I'm also talking about you.

Here are all the things I like about the food system as it is:

• For me, at my income, food is always there when I am hungry. I almost never have to think about whether I will eat, just what and where and when.

Case in point: deep into week three I woke after a late afternoon nap hungry and cold. When you live alone no one has been cooking and baking while you sleep. You have to deal. The sun had gone down while I was sleeping, so the day's heat had dissipated. I needed something fast and filling and zippy to eat. In the good old days—just three weeks earlier—I would have started with chocolate—cranking the brain over with some high-octane sugar and choco-caffeine. Then I would have headed for carbs—comfort food. Now there was nothing I could nuke. No Chinese takeout. No day-old burrito. No bread for toast. I did manage, of course. I actually whipped up a hot soup by boiling potatoes and carrots, sautéing leeks, herbs, and garlic, and throwing it all in a blender; it took twenty minutes from feet hitting floor to spoon entering mouth. It hit the spot—but some good industrial system cookies would have been a bull's-eye.

• I don't have to think much about food at all—my mind is free to roam in higher planes of thought. I don't have to spend half my day getting it, either.
• Food is someone else's problem. What it takes to get it to the supermarket, nicely packaged, never has to be any of my business, and Lord knows I have a lot of business that *is* mine. We'd never have gotten a man on the moon or personal computers if everyone had to grow their own.
• The global marketplace means that I can get my bananas from India if crops fail in Thailand, and I don't have to think for a second about that switch. The anonymity of my supplier allows me to ignore the plights of farmers far away. I don't subscribe to this—I just notice how easy the system makes it for me to ignore it.
• I have choices galore. Exotic and everyday cheese. Wholesome and Yaya bread. Several dozen cuts of meat packaged and sometimes

even spiced. Store-brand to high-end brands of teas and coffees. Condiments. Soups. Oils. Nut butters. Spices. Canned and boxed foods with pretty labels. Juices. Cereals. Crackers. Cookies. I really— like, *really*—don't want to give any of this up.

• I have fruit and vegetables no matter what the season. Those bins are never bare.

• Deli counters are laden with creamy, savory, attractive, tart, sweet, pungent, complex prepared salads and quiches and Yuppie burritos with olives, feta, avocado, and such. Aah, and those wonderful roast chickens with three different flavoring mixes.

• I can indulge in every kind of flavor and texture I want any day of the week. There are eight restaurants in Langley alone. Go twenty miles north or east and I can have Thai, Indian, Ethiopian, Vietnamese, Japanese, and more.

• By and large, I can afford to buy what I want. Especially if I stock up during sales.

• With rare exceptions I don't have to wonder if the food will kill me. I may worry if the accumulation of one of those thirty ingredients in prepared foods will kill me in the long run, but rarely do I have to worry if the can in my hand is full of botulism, which would kill me right away.

• Finally (and you'll notice it's last), there is the moral issue. Doesn't industrial food do some good? Doesn't it feed the world? Doesn't it fill food banks? Isn't having my cake (chips, crackers, nuts, etc.) balanced by the poor and hungry having at the very least their rice too? If we disconnect from this global food system, don't we doom millions of people to death by starvation, by a kind of hunger beyond anything I've experienced, the kind that kills more than ten thousand people a year?

This last point seals the deal for me, but not without misgivings. The industrial system stays, not just because it suits me but because we still need it to feed the world. Despite how it depletes and poisons the land. Despite how much fossil fuel it requires. Despite how egregious it seems to patent and modify the genetic code of the very seeds of life. Despite the way Big Farm is muscling out small farmers around the world. Despite it all, this system generally still supplies ample, available, cheap, and safe food. And we don't yet have an alternative that can do the same. Even shoppers at the upscale organic Whole Foods (which food activists call Whole Paycheck) have to face that little is from small local farmers; more than eight thousand acres of greenhouses in Mexico produce much of our winter supply, along with the Florida tomatoes that famously exploit cheap labor.

I was giving myself a lecture that was part preference, part realism, and part parroting what I'd been told. Yet I didn't like it.

My blog posts during the third week were mostly cheerful and inventive, even when I'd report on something disturbing, like the food riots in Mozambique because the Russian wheat crop had failed. Still, I was groping. I was haunted by the question I'd posed to Pam Mitchell that got me on this crazy track: Can we, the people of Whidbey, feed ourselves from Whidbey? In essence, she had scoffed at the idea. Even our best efforts are a pittance, she said, and require the global system to persist.

Let me give you an example of the need for industrial agriculture. We have a food bank, Good Cheer, that is supported by the sales from their two thrift stores where I regularly look for bargains to stock my kitchen and clothes closets for pennies. In the process I am also feeding the coffers that feed the tummies and soul of the community. We are enormously proud of the respectful and effective programs of Good Cheer, but . . . only a small percentage of the food distributed is local. Last year five thousand pounds of vegetables came out of the food bank's organic garden or from donations from gleaners, farmers' market vendors, home gardeners, and such, but far more comes from

1. Food Lifeline, the regional food pantry supplier. Through their own independent efforts, fierce deals are struck with large suppliers. Industrial food. At a fraction of what we pay at the grocery store.

2. food drives by businesses, churches, and organizations. These yield thousands of pounds of canned and boxed goods a year—all of it industrial.

3. donations of nearly outdated but still good produce, baked goods, dairy products, and other goods from local grocers, which are still primarily industrial food.

How could we feed our community's hungry without industrial food? That question bothered me. A lot. Later I saw that it was not the right question, but for the nonce it flew in the face of local as a way of eating.

My Neighbor the Local Berry Farmer Turned Global Food Expert

In the meanwhile, I needed to find someone who could help me figure out whether Whidbey really could someday be self-sufficient in food. That's when I recalled a meeting several years ago where a group of farmers, chefs, and entrepreneurs got together to understand one another and how we are connected.

Gene Kahn was one of the local speakers. He lives on the island now—in Coupeville—but he used to be an organic berry farmer in Skagit Valley until he scaled up his operation, developed the Cascadian brand, and sold it to General Mills. He then went on to work in numerous capacities on international sustainability initiatives, including as senior adviser for Agricultural Development at the Bill & Melinda Gates Foundation. While he looks like the rest of us—fleece and jeans—he's a world-class expert who brings a much larger lens to the local food question.

Gene stirred up a hornet's nest at that meeting by goading the small-scale CSA and market gardeners to graduate from dirt farming or die. Turn your produce into jams, chutneys, chips, pies, canned, dried and frozen fruits and vegetables, he said, because that is where the money is. You don't want to be a supplier. You want to be a producer. And then you want to scale up. Vertically integrate. Develop markets beyond the island.

Fur and feathers flew. He was challenging our commitment to local food and local economies. People didn't like it, and Gene didn't like being the brunt of their aversion to big.

Even though I am habitually on the side of the little guy, I never forgot Gene's challenge. As I sought a middle-ground food ethic between purist and pragmatist, I decided to visit him to get his take on this question that was growing in my mind: Without the industrial food system, could we on Whidbey Island eat?

I drove twenty-five miles north to Coupeville, turned up his long drive, and parked by his small house. He'd instructed me to come around to the barn, which looked like . . . well, a barn. Once inside, it was a different story. In a side room he had several impeccably refinished vintage cars in an immaculate tile-floored "garage." Even my food-sensitive friends would have eaten off that floor. Gene led me through the unfinished part of the barn, up a flight of stairs, and into his office.

Gene collected original editions of books about farming, agriculture, and gardening even more passionately than he did his restored vintage cars. He had what looked like miles of floor-to-ceiling shelves, every shelf dusted, every book lined up, with frailer ones in plastic pouches. His desk was clear. He had two bottles of Perrier on the coffee table in front of a leather couch and chair. He had clearly moved far from his roots as a hippie in the seventies—but had not left his altruism and compassion behind.

When I asked Gene whether people on Whidbey could feed themselves, he looked at me as if I were a freshman who'd asked the ultimate dumb question. Which, quite honestly, I deserved. I know I was and still am a novice on this subject of feeding even myself, much less the island or the world. But the answer from the hardheaded businessman gave me hope. According to Gene, feeding Whidbey wasn't hard at all. But, he told me, I hadn't really asked the right question.

He went on to point out that the prairie that runs across the center of our island—and is now protected from development as a historical and farming reserve—covers nearly eighteen thousand acres. Put that all in vegetables and we can do it. The problem is that farmers don't want to. They're independent, and they've been farming for years. They aren't going to be told what to grow. Furthermore, people won't put up with a diet of only what can grow here—potatoes, squash, beans, greens, and brassicas. Throw in some fish, chicken, and beef—but less than we're used to—and you still have a pretty boring diet. We are all diehard individualists in a free country. We want to do, have, and eat what we want.

Gene Kahn isn't even interested in this question, though. His job with the Gates Foundation requires him to think about the people in Africa who are starving to death, who have been largely robbed of their subsistence way of life, who live in poverty in cities or in desperation in drought-devastated rural villages. He thinks about the poor here as well, who need cheap food in order to manage. To think local, to him, is to forget these people. To consign them to starvation while we, the well heeled, feed ourselves.

The problem with the local or organic idealists, he seemed to say, is that they aren't thinking about the road from where we are (99 percent industrial) to where we want to be (a variety of food sources). Yes, ideally, all food would be local, organic, plentiful, and affordable (likely setting us back more than the 8 percent of budget we now spend on food, but less than the 31 percent of budget we spent in the 1950s). But how do we get there?

Kahn isn't rejecting small-scale agriculture. He's rejecting it as a scalable alternative to a science-based, politically achievable, and adequate food and fiber system . . . at least for the foreseeable future. Eventually it would be ideal if all food was organic, ethical, and supportive of local economies, but to get there you have to effectively solve for every variable in the whole food-supply chain: seeds, inputs, pest management, weeding, harvesting, processing, packaging, shipping, distributing, and educating the eater to want this alternative. I gleaned some important insights from his bigger food system view.

Fertility

In an interview published in *Fast Company*[2] when Kahn was still at General Mills, the company that owned his Cascadian brand, he said, "We'd need to find organic sources for a whole host of nutrients. The best, the most practical way would be to build a whole new composting infrastructure across the United States. That would require tremendous coordination across municipalities, and much more thorough composting of all human refuse."

Could he possibly be talking about poop? Gene pulled from a bottom shelf, in a plastic protective sleeve, a copy of the book that had become a provocative reference for me in my back-to-the-land days: F. H. (Franklin Hiram) King, *Farmers of Forty Centuries*. The key to their long survival? "Night soil." Composted poop.

That poop (or humanure, as it is called now) might save us inspired me to add to my food system to-do list. Item 7: Get organic matter out of the waste stream and landfills and put it back in the soil.

Scalability

When the *Fast Company* interviewer posed the question of whether local organic can scale up, Gene's view was that "it's going to happen incrementally . . . to imagine that we were going to change U.S. agriculture and keep it all in the hands of market gardeners, instead of production scale farmers, is not only a fatuous dream, it's an undesirable perspective from my view. . . . I think [change is] happening. But . . . we'll make sure this gets done right and done in a way that is really sustainable. . . . The conversation . . . should be about how we change the world for the better, how we deal with the world as we currently see it. Not about creating some impossible dream.

"And that's what's critical: the improvement. Whether we get to

100% organic is not the issue. It's whether we become a sustainable society."

Gene was not saying that what is best for people and planet is impossible. He just said it will take time, and needs to be well thought through and "sold" to people at every link of the food chain. It won't be a case of either/or, or purist versus industrialist, but rather a process to change from the world as it presents itself to us now to the world we want.

I left with a lot to chew on, so to speak. As I drove back home I started to put together a framework I could swallow. I see now that the task of change is far more complex than a one-size-fits-all solution. Despite my own experiment I don't expect everyone on Whidbey to go 100 percent local. We'd scrape this place clean of food in short order.

As Gene points out, the pathways need to be evolutionary, not revolutionary. I can personally run radical experiments and propose radical shifts, but society and even nature don't work that way. They evolve over time. Our visionaries—prophets and revolutionaries—jolt us awake. But our innovators, engineers, architects, and educators actually build the future incrementally over time.

From the conversation with Gene and my own struggle to understand the bigger picture, a goal I could believe in started to coalesce.

I don't want to promote an end product; I want to map a path. That path would go all the way from our food psychology, culture, and preferences to growing some of our own to eating what our market gardeners grow to regional eating to a healthier global food system.

The map would make sense, be clear, feel empowering, and get people laughing as well as motivated.

Eventually I'd understand how truly complex this is, weaving sovereignty and security and affordability and availability and safety and sustainability and delight all into one fabric. But for now, I was just excited about the prospect of looking more closely at the entire world of food.

Clearly I needed to finish my 10-mile diet with integrity, start planning for my 50/50 February caper, and then see whatever lies beyond that next big mountain.

Now It's Your Turn

As you can tell, it took some considerable effort to reconcile myself to the limitations of local. Here are some tips and practices for your own adaptations in terms of cost, quantity, and kind of food.

Conscious Eating

Globally, the food-industrial complex pumps out more than twenty-seven hundred calories a day for every man, woman, and child[3]—in the United States it's closer to four thousand[4]—and yet, despite areas of malnutrition, 30 to 50 percent of the world's food goes to waste. It is way too easy to take food for granted, load up plates, and go from famished to bloated without even noticing "full." Here are some tips that help prevent overeating:

80 Percent

Eat until you are 80 percent full. Okinawans are among the longest-lived people on the earth, and one of their secrets is *hara hachi bu*, the rule of eating until you are 80 percent full. If you are out of touch with full, you might need to slow down your eating until you actually feel that one more bite would be too much. Knowing full, you can feel 80 percent; for me that means I have to pause between bites to check in with my stomach.

One trick I use: I commit to leaving one bite on my plate. Aware of that last bite, I am mindful through the first dozen bites, the mind checking for whether I'm close to the end. Otherwise, I could find myself done before consciousness begins.

Shrink Your Plate Size

A recent study found that plate size affects how much we eat. In 1900 the average dinner plate was nine inches wide. By 1950 plates had grown to ten inches. Now they are closer to twelve inches. It's hard to judge proper portion size when the plate's so big. Our brains understand portion in terms of proportion—how much of the plate is filled, how big a serving spoon is used.

Learning this got me wondering . . . is the size of our girth related to the size of our dishes? In 1950, 9.7 percent of the U.S. population was obese and now it's 34 percent.

Does the lower relative cost of industrial food trick us into eating more? In 1950, we spent a third of our income on food. Now, according to the USDA,[5] overall Americans spend less than 10 percent of their income on food (though if you make less than twenty thousand dollars a year you join the global middle class, spending about 25 percent).

So now I use my big dinner plates for heaping salads and steamed greens. For the rest I use the next size down.

When I backslide into late-night "barefoot in front of open fridge with spoon in hand," I can break the spell by taking out one of my three-inch saucers, heaping it high with six almonds and twenty raisins, and paddling back to my office indulged.

Savor Your Food

Take pleasure in the flavors and see how long you can still taste your food before swallowing. Focus on how the mouthful tastes as you chew. The old fuddy-duddy rule of thumb is twenty chews for each bite. My trick: savor the flavor as long as possible. Interestingly, meat loses its flavor sooner than other whole foods—at least in my mouth.

Slow Down

Whether you want to savor your food or notice when you are full, slowing down helps. Two ways I do this are putting my fork down between bites (my generation was taught that as manners) and dining with friends with the intention of being leisurely.

Track Your Daily Bread

Write down everything you eat each day. Not to count calories but to be aware of your own hand-to-mouth habits. You could think of it as savoring your food a second time—when you review your eating day. Such tracking will naturally reveal unconscious eating.

Try a Whole-Foods Lent

Like my friend Suzanne, you could engage in a whole-foods Lent— forty days of nothing packaged, prepared, or processed. After a few days of calculating what she'd eaten and a few more negotiating with the butcher to sell her meat wrapped in paper rather than shrink-wrapped, she did fine. The Lenten practice was less about her preferences and more about how whole-foods eaters interface with a highly-processed-foods culture.

Change Your Relationship to Meat

Vegetarians argue for no-meat diets on the grounds of personal and environmental health, longevity, and cruelty-free eating. Many others argue for meat eating: Atkins, Paleo, Abascal, and Weston Price diets have meat as a key element. My 10-mile diet showed me a middle ground based on learning what it takes to pasture-raise animals and an understanding of how livestock is part of most well-managed small farms. Pastured animals fertilize pastures as they graze; provide manure for biodynamic preparations; and feed family, friends, and communities milk, butter, cheese, eggs, and flesh. Choosing to eat only locally grown pastured animals will naturally slow down your meat consumption. The supply isn't endless and the price is appropriate to the work invested and the dignity of the animal.

Here are some explorations and practices around the issue of meat:

MEAT AS A TREAT

Track how much meat you eat in a normal week. Be honest. Don't skimp because you're watching. Get that hot grocery store chicken if you love it. Order ahi tuna. Grab a Whopper. Whatever is part of your weekly meat routine.

10 PERCENT RULE

Use the 10 percent rule to moderate that. If you eat 40 ounces of meat a week, for example, go for 36. If that seems plenty, drop it to 32 ounces. Keep it up, slowly, until you cut into your true appetite for meat. Then add an ounce and stabilize there. As I've said, I started at about 45 ounces and now eat about 20. I eat an occasional juicy steak for my inner carnivore, though I now find I'll box half the restaurant portion and make it last a few days.

MEATLESS MONDAY

The Meatless Monday campaign was designed to help people eschew chewing meat one day a week. It's like the old Catholic fish on Friday—a habit in service to a set of beliefs. It's a choice that affects many things at once: weight, health, justice, sustainability, climate disruption, rainforest preservation, and your grandchildren's future. If you were told you could take a pill that would have all these effects, you'd do it. Less meat is no bitter pill.

SUNDAY DINNER

Roll back the clock to an era when we ate a Sunday roast that became Monday sandwiches and Tuesday spaghetti sauce and Wednesday tacos and Thursday soup, followed by a couple of days of macaroni and cheese, leading to another extraordinary Sunday dinner.

EAT HALF

Set aside half your meat at the beginning of a restaurant meal. Bring your own container or ask for ones made of compostable material. Voilà! Another meal.

DO IT YOURSELF

Participate in slaughtering and butchering an animal at least once in your life. If you've never done it, you'll have a searing experience, making meat either unpalatable or holy or primal.

The No-Meat Mantra

Say again and again: "Nuts and seeds [beans, sesame, pumpkin, sunflower] are protein; nuts and seeds are protein" until the grip of the cultural indoctrination about animal products being the only source of protein is gone. In fact, most vegetables are high in amino acids.

All of these both objectively run less meat through your body and interrupt your behavior patterns so that you can rechoose how much you need or want to eat.

Hint!

Relocalizing your food is easier if you try to eat whole foods—that is, foods with only one ingredient, like any fruit or vegetable, plain meat or fish, whole grains, beans, nuts, and plain dairy.

Try These Recipes

After all the talk of chicken, it's time for a delicious recipe from Patrick Boin of The Braeburn, for chicken served up with his essential ingredient: integrity. But first here's one of Georgie Smith's traditional central Whidbey farming community recipes.

Farmer Georgie Smith is carrying on the heritage of her four-generation family farm, Willowood Farm of Ebey's Prairie. Her great-grandfather settled here in the late 1800s and farmed the rich prairie soil of Central Whidbey. Over the years the farm grew grains, peas, iris bulbs, sheep, winter squash, cattle, and a great love of the land and the farm. Farmer Georgie today grows twelve acres of mixed fresh market vegetables, selling to local Whidbey Island farmers' markets and to restaurants in Island, Skagit, and King counties that are committed to using local foods. Farmer Georgie works hand in hand with her father (he is in charge of all the equipment!) and has high hopes that her two young daughters will one day carry on in her farming footsteps.

⁂

Nutty Renee's Red Kuri Soup

Named in honor of my mother, Renee, who came up with this recipe featuring the rich, hazelnut-reminiscent flavor of red kuri winter squash. Peanut butter brings out the creamy sweetness of the squash, but be careful to not overdo it as the peanut can also easily overpower the delicate flavors.

2 cups red kuri squash from a 2-pound squash, roasted
2 cups chicken stock
1 tablespoon olive oil
½ cup pine nuts
¼ cup finely chopped onion
½ cup milk
1 tablespoon freshly ground pepper
¼ cup (no more) quality peanut butter (like Adams)
Baby spinach leaves or arugula, for garnish

Cut the red kuri squash in half, scoop out the seeds, and roast it until it's soft. Roasting the squash is important as it partially caramelizes the vegetable, which is great for the flavors. Let it cool and then scoop out the flesh. In a food processor, add the chicken stock and squash and puree until smooth.

In a large saucepan, heat the olive oil, then sauté the pine nuts and onion until soft. Let cool and then chop coarsely (in the food processor if possible). Transfer back to the pot, add the squash, and simmer the entire mixture.

Fifteen minutes before serving, add the milk, pepper, and peanut butter and stir well. Do not boil after this step.

Garnish with the baby spinach leaves or arugula and serve. Other squash or pumpkins can be substituted, but be sure to roast them!

Patrick Boin at The Braeburn says:

> As for a personal philosophy toward cooking and why I do what I do, I am a steward for the earth and all she provides. I have a responsibility to the planet, my community, the local farms and farmers who work them, and my coworkers to prepare this bounty with humility, respect, honor, and grace. I am a simple man making my way through the universe, and kitchen groovin' is my ride of choice.

Chanterelle and Cauliflower Mushroom—Stuffed Roasted Chicken Breast

Two 6-ounce boneless, skinless chicken breasts
2 tablespoons cold-pressed extra virgin olive oil
¼ cup Romanesco cauliflower
1 teaspoon capers
1 tablespoon minced fresh garlic (2 cloves)
2 tablespoons diced red onion, small dice
1 ounce cooking sherry
1 ounce white wine
1 cup chanterelle mushrooms, cleaned and torn
1 cup cauliflower mushrooms, cleaned and torn
1 teaspoon finely chopped fresh rosemary

2 tablespoons finely chopped fresh parsley

1 teaspoon chopped fresh sage, fine chiffonade

1 teaspoon stemmed fresh thyme

¼ cup Craisins

½ teaspoon sea salt

½ teaspoon freshly cracked black pepper

¼ cup panko bread crumbs

¼ cup water

1 ounce butter

Preheat the oven to 400°F and adjust a rack to the middle position.

Wash the chicken breasts, remove excess fat and tendons, pat them dry, and lay them flat. At the meaty part make an incision and split the chicken nearly in two, leaving a ¼-inch "spine" on the back side. Cover and set them aside in the refrigerator.

Heat the oil in a medium sauté pan just to the smoking point, then add the Romanesco cauliflower, capers, garlic, and onion. Turn the heat to medium.

Sauté over medium heat for 2 minutes, then add ½ ounce each of the sherry and the wine; continue to sauté for 2 minutes.

Bring the heat up to high, then add the mushrooms, rosemary, parsley, sage, thyme, and Craisins; continue to sauté for another 3 minutes, adding the remaining sherry and wine in the last minute.

Remove the mixture from the heat and place it in a small mixing bowl, add the salt, pepper, and panko, and incorporate with a light hand.

Remove the chicken breasts from the refrigerator, lay them flat, and open them so you have a "butterfly"; fill one side of each breast with half the stuffing, then cover with the opposite flap; gently pat any remaining filling on the top of the breasts.

Place the breasts in a small baking dish, add the water and butter, cover with a piece of foil, and bake in the preheated oven for 30 minutes.

Remove from the oven and check the temperature (the internal center reading should be 165°F).

Plate with a quinoa salad and life is sublime.

Notes

no sweatshop chicken

size matters—bigger takes longer

use mushrooms that inspire you; their earthiness will always shine
    through

be seasonal with your vegetables

adjustments may be necessary

most important . . . make this recipe yours; after all, it's for you—peace

CHAPTER SEVEN

Revelations of the Final Week

Home stretch! I could almost smell October 1 like a horse smells the stable. In Spanish they call it *querencia*—a wonderful word for that longing we feel, when stressed, for home or turf, stable or lair—for that place where we rest and gather strength. After a long ride, *querencia* fuels a last burst as the worn-out horse gallops to the barn.

In week four, my *querencia* was toast. With cheese. And certainly nuts.

I actually made a list of my sweet (and salty and oily) weak spots, the "eating-home" I yearned for:

- chocolate-covered almonds
- a handful of nuts a day
- nonwheat bread
- cheese—but really good cheese as a flavor, not a food
- dried fruit—prunes, apricots, raisins, figs, peaches
- Mr. Mobley's sauce (a Whidbey delicacy) and/or goddess salad dressing
- almond butter
- stevia! (my natural alternative to artificial sweeteners)

Once written, that list seemed too short. Surely I'd need avocados. And crackers, three types. And rice and oatmeal. And . . .

At the same time, the constraints of September had wrung some precious insights out of me, and I wasn't about to toss those out once

I opened the door again to the Industrial Cornucopia. I occupied myself in this last week with long journal entries and blog posts on the big picture of my very little picture of local eating. For me, seeing patterns and systems is almost as yummy as toast with melted cheese, so I relished—so to speak—this chance to mull it all over.

As I reflected on what had changed, I saw three levels: the objective report, the practical changes, and the spiritual tempering.

We'll start with the facts. The tallies and measurements. I totaled it all up and posted the following:

Ladies and Gentlemen, the Tallies Are In

I know you are waiting with bated breath to get the results of this month of 10-mile eating. Here are some highlights:

Weight: I lost six pounds. My average calories a day were 1,600 so that accounts for some of it. I'll bet that without grains I lost water weight—no swelling in hands and feet.

Cholesterol: Tricia's part of the bargain was to feed me. My part of the bargain, beyond not cheating, was to get my blood work done before and after the 10-mile diet experiment. So here's the numbers:

Total cholesterol down 3
HDL (good) up 7
LDL (bad) down 9
Risk ratio from 4.2 (about average) to 3.7 (low range)

These are the kind of numbers in a month that the doc says, "Whatever you are doing, keep doing it."

Calories: Fifty percent of the calories came from Tricia (supplemented by my garden and some extras from friends). That's good news, bad news.

Good news is: Wow! That's a lot of food grown by the one little industrious Tricia.

The bad news is that without the extra milk, meat, honey, oil, and a little cheese, I'd have been definitely underfed.

Ahh, but the good news is, ALL the food except for the oil, salt, caffeine, and 30 little limes came from my 10 miles. That is very, very hopeful in terms of our ability to feed ourselves.

Ahh, but the bad news is that everyone who wants to eat this way would need to grow a big kitchen garden with plenty of squash and potatoes, and (except vegans) would need to at least be part of a chicken and goat/cow coop OR form a relationship with a grower who can provide this. Our current CSA and agricultural production couldn't feed us all—all year. Yet.

The good news is that just beyond my 10 miles up on Ebey's Prairie, people are growing grains and beans, and if there were more demand for such, I'm sure more land would be put into those crops. We do not need to do without bread! Or beans in our winter soups.

The bad news is that demographically we are an aging population, and if we don't find a way to attract and retain young farmers we will not be able to feed ourselves into our dotage.

The overall news is that we are actually on our way to at least partial food self sufficiency on the island if we would eat what we can grow here—and not insist on what cannot grow here. And if we commit to support our producers by buying from them, especially during the transition as an integrated food system develops here. And if we are wise about what we need from 100 miles and 300 miles and 1000 miles—we actually can map our food system against our food needs—and begin to actually address the challenge Pam set before us and all eat more than one month a year.

Taking Stock

For the sake of the grand experiment, Tricia and I kept track of the food she gave me and the food I acquired within (and beyond) my ten miles. I ate nearly 50,000 calories that month. Sounds like a lot when you think in terms of days, but divided by 30 that's about 1,650 a day. A tenth of that total was milk! Half was meat and eggs. I drank three cups of oil for 3,500 calories, and two and a half cups of honey for 2,500.

All this is sobering on two accounts. One is that I eat a lot. I can start to see how I'll die having passed six tons of food through my alimentary canal. The other is that without my exotics and 10-mile extras, I would have consumed only 750 calories a day. You can see why it takes a complete food system to feed a village—not industrial monocrops, not just backyard vegetables. Later, in February, I would add grains and beans. With those I could have had adequate calories without any animal products, but even so, I saw the level of focus and intention it would take to feed the villages of Whidbey from the farms and ranches of Whidbey—and that much would need to change to make food a shared priority.

Then I assessed the changes I'd made and thought would last.

They say you create a new habit by faithfully doing it for twenty-one days. Indeed. The 10-mile diet had settled into a routine, and I was satisfied with it. In twenty-one days I'd turned my cooking and eating around. I had

- restocked my kitchen with local foods.
- learned to cook formerly overlooked foods, like turnips and kohl-rabi.
- pulled out my old pressure cooker and Foley food mill and put them to work.
- learned what it takes to make flour and would forevermore bless the hands that grow, harvest, thresh, grind, and package what before seemed a lowly food, best consumed as sourdough toast.
- learned to make zackers and zookies, though I was sure I'd revert to toast on October 1.
- learned to make butter, which went from miracle in week one to standard practice by now.
- developed not just a tolerance of but a real taste for raw milk and ultrafresh greens, and truly free-range chicken—worth every penny.

- come to savor my food more because I knew what it took to grow it.
- come to love my farmers, not just "know them," as food activists suggest.

I had also rekindled my love of writing. At first the blog posts felt like a guilty pleasure. I had more important things to do. Every day, though, had been a revelation. Each insight made me hungry for the next, and for telling my readers what I'd learned. Readers? The blog had one follower at the beginning: Tricia. By the end of the month, though, *Yes!* magazine reposted the pick of the week's litter to their weekly distribution list. I was reading my food dictionary daily and watching TED talks and documentaries, all the while presuming that this was a trifling sideline. I was like a committed bachelorette who'd stumbled into a relationship with the milquetoast in the apartment next door. Hmmm. Milk toast. Another food from childhood.

Retox

Even so, I presumed it would be a romance, not a marriage. I had no pretentions of changing my diet for good, but I wondered what would stick. Might I need some new guidelines once I took off the 10-mile corset, promises to myself about behaviors that would anchor the transformations when the tides turned and the old foods flooded my life? Here's what I went on to write:

I suspect I will never lose sight of my food system, and will weigh the source of a product—and the possibility of local substitution—as I shop.

I suspect I will now invest more dollars in my local food system—as a shopper and as an investor and as a donor. I know I can get factory-farmed chicken for ⅓ what I pay a local grower (i.e. friend), but I'd rather buy meat from my neighbors if possible. There is a principle called subsidiarity: Meet needs as close to home/source as possible and only go further afield if the solution isn't at hand. Yes, I do want to eat local meat, and if I eat less because it costs more, that's approved behavior in a range of diets. If I can't get local, well, I'll get regional.

I suspect I will also buy fair-trade products that aren't grown anywhere near me. Tea and coffee. Chocolate. I want to support local whether it is mine or a coffee bean grower in Colombia or Kenya. Relational eating and fair eating mean supporting farmers everywhere in staying on their land. Which isn't easy for them, because subsistence and sustainable farming is very, very hard work.

I suspect I will grow a very different garden next year. I have been a hobby gardener. Put some seeds in the ground and shout hallelujah if anything but kale and zucchini flourishes. I think I can plan a rotation for my four beds to produce more substantial and plentiful food. More carrots and beans. More herbs (rosemary, basil and oregano in enough quantity to dry for winter). Fennel for flavor. Beets, turnips and rutabagas to store for the winter. Potatoes. Potatoes. Potatoes. I'll get the winter squash in earlier so I will hopefully get more than three of them. I'd like to try parsnips too. And Roma tomatoes that are good for sauce. As for fruit, I now know I want an apple tree and an Italian plum tree. We just must have sweet.

Of course for very good reason I'll have lots of kale and zucchini and patty pan squash. That reason being—if all else fails, I have something from the soil.

The Missing Ingredient

Yet something was still missing from my local formula. What was it? I smacked my lips together as if my tongue were tasting for the elusive flavor.

Aah! People. Where were the people around the table in this new ethic of relational eating. Like so many of us solo people in our culture, I'd gotten used to solitary dining.

Eating alone was the downside of living alone, a state I love after thirty-five years of living cheek by jowl with a bunch of other people. The quiet. The dominion over my choices. Being the mistress of my time. Taking in only the chatter I choose through e-mail, phone calls, and my trips down into Langley for food, mail, and conversation.

It turns out that I am not alone—so to speak. Solo living is an up-and-coming lifestyle. There are more than 32 million of us free to dine with a spoon in front of the fridge.

Families don't fare that much better. Less than 60 percent of families with teens manage even five sit-down dinners together a week. Research shows that family dinners do a world of good, positively affecting grades, reducing stress, improving nutrition, and cutting the risk of getting into drugs, smoking, or drinking. But even so, we can't seem to get ourselves on the same schedule.

Eric Klinenberg in his book *Going Solo* points out that in 1950, less than 10 percent of households were singles. Now 28 percent—and rising—of households are singles. In most cities, that goes up to nearly 40 percent. In New York City it's 50 percent. Apparently this is what happens in countries with rising incomes, a good social-safety net, and greater economic independence for women. Population experts have learned that the best way to drive down births is to give women economic independence. Now we're seeing that going to another level, with millions of women, like me, discovering they like to be quirky— and alone. My friends still reassure me, "Don't worry, you'll meet someone," as if my solitude were a burden. Even when I've "met someone," I never thought it would be fun to have them underfoot.

But come dinnertime I always feel odd. Where are the other people around the table? After thirty-five years in community with a family dinner at 6:30 every night, eating without savoring conversation is not as nourishing.

I wondered how this 10-mile diet might affect my solo eating—if I would now broaden out again to feeding others, to breaking bread. Why, besides living alone, did I not share meals with other?

Busy Day, Busy Day, No Time to Make a Friend

I—like the majority of my friends and many families, apparently— am busy, busy, busy. I don't even have time for inviting friends, it seems, much less preparing a meal for them. Unknown minions in kitchens and factories cook for us. Prepackaged meals and take-out meals allow us all to eat without cooking. Putting dinner on the table is as quick as calling for pizza or buying a preroasted chicken at the market. It's less of a social occasion. Is it also more of an overeating occasion? Certainly I tend to eat more when no one is watching. Do others? Is there any correlation between living alone and obesity?

Back in the hunter-gatherer days, being ostracized was tantamount to being executed. We needed one another to survive. We still do, but the fact is hidden behind that *Wizard of Oz* screen of self-sufficiency. We wouldn't last much more than a week without our farmers, whatever the scale of their operations, yet we eat almost as if going to the industrial outlet called "the market" magically produces food!

Is this a victory or a loss? Just because humans once needed their tribes to survive in the hunter-gatherer days doesn't mean that eating together makes us human. Or does it? Are we by nature convivial—social creatures who flourish by sharing the vicissitudes of living? I wanted to come back to the tribe before the 10-mile diet was done. I wanted to welcome people into my 10-mile culture, to affirm the sufficiency and deliciousness of my food by feeding another. And who better than Tricia!

The Last Supper?

I was a rusty hostess—my meals and home arranged around solitude—but it was time to reciprocate my feeder's generosity by feeding her. For more than a month Tricia had filled both my heart and my belly. I wanted my last official 10-mile supper to be with her and her husband, Kent, and I knew just what to serve. One of Tobey's 10-mile twenty-five-dollar chickens.

On September 30 I scrubbed, swept, and vacuumed to a higher standard than I hold for just myself, and filled the house with the perfume of home cooking.

Tricia and Kent showed up all smiles and with a few extra vegetables since we'd developed such a momma-and-baby-bird relationship. Kent has a round face that lights up when he smiles, and had always seemed to me a man with enthusiasm to spare. Whenever we'd been at a meeting together he'd nearly bounced up out of his chair to offer at least two or three inventive solutions to any problem we encountered. When I first met Tricia in the choir, there had been no Kent on the horizon. Now they were work as well as life partners, Tricia the gardener, Kent—by day a teacher—the builder of fences and sheds and greenhouses.

Soon we were at the table for the meal. I'd roasted the chicken with Tricia's garlic and rosemary inserted under the skin and inside the cavity for flavor. I'd also roasted some of Tricia's vegetables: onions, potatoes, turnips (aah, how I love them now), and carrots. For the salad (Tricia's greens, tomatoes, and cucumbers) I made a dressing of crushed garlic, fresh chopped basil and oregano, and those precious exotics, oil and lime juice. For dessert I'd cored some of Tricia's apples, drizzled Island Apiaries' honey in the wells, and baked them. I put out a pitcher of Belinda's cream for the apples and the coffee and tea.

We carved the chicken as though it were a Thanksgiving turkey, slicing the breast meat rather than just serving a whole breast to one person, a leg and thigh to another. Maybe it was the slow, rich, ambling conversation, maybe as food producers we were all viscerally aware of what it took to put that meal on the table, maybe the meat itself was more filling and tasty because the bird had had a happy life out in the grass, pecking at grubs and organic feed. Whatever, there were actually leftovers that I portioned out over days, making the price per meal equal to wolfing down a miserable, grown-in-the-dark, beak-clipped, factory-farmed bird in two sittings. Alone.

Our conversation delved below the level of food and farming to how Tricia and Kent met, fell in love, and married, and then deeper to our spiritual beliefs and experiences. It was then that I learned of Kent's mystical bent and his study of Rudolf Steiner—biodynamic farming and a whole body of work on the integration of nature, spirit, and daily life. I'd never had a chance to learn firsthand about Steiner's thoughts and we talked long into the night.

All the while a warmth spread in my belly that was the opposite of hunger. It was the fullness of giving.

In India they say, "The guest is God." By feeding Tricia and Kent I was paying forward all the cups of warm beverages and little empañadas and cheeses and fruit and even Coca-Colas I'd received in homes across this world. I returned to the tribe—if only for an evening. I realized how I need people just as much as I need crunch or chocolate or calories. Local is a place in the heart as well as one way to fill my stomach. Like that moment in my backyard when food became where I belonged, not just what I bought, this dinner reminded me that feeding and being fed makes us belong to one another, makes us a people.

I went to bed so very satisfied, body and soul.

I slept. I woke. And it was . . .

October 1

Toast! It was such an event, I wrote it large in my journal. Followed by:

Crunch!

I topped the toast with almond butter and sat down to eat it with my standard tea, honey, and milk, cat on my lap, journal on the arm of the chair, feet up, eyes gazing at the beautiful line of fir trees to the east of my house and Mt. Baker to the north.

I made it. Yet it made me too. Or remade me. Besides having lost six pounds, something different was simmering in my soul. My friend, author, and global activist Lynne Twist, said once, "We don't do our projects. We enter them and they transform us."

What had changed within me? I asked and waited for answers to come, jotting them in my journal.

Homecoming

The first thought that came was this: Now I know I live somewhere.

I've lived in houses in towns and cities, yes, but I'd never cast my lot so fully with a place and a people, with the local farmers, farms, fields, forest, and friends who live here too. In Rhinelander I'd learned to grow a garden, butcher animals, and process food, but we were isolated from town, and we relied less on our garden than on our burlap bags of rice, beans, and potatoes. While I wasn't sure "we"—as in all of us here on the island—could live "here" as religiously as I had this month, I knew that my effort to do so had knitted me into the community at a most profound level. A real community of place where people with differences live together and find common ground.

Where had I been living before September, anyway?

With perfect postmodern irony I thought, I live in my mind. A skin-encapsulated, life-process animated bundle of thoughts. A child of Descartes' "I think, therefore I am." The "I-that-thinks" has actually been the only consistent address for what I call me. Born in Oklahoma, I lived sixteen years on Long Island before I was off and running. Rhode Island, Madrid, and Brooklyn formed a six-year runway to taking off for parts unknown. I then spent fifteen years "on the road"—on and off living in a motor home punctuated by stints in driveways and rental homes for projects in Mexico, Arizona, Wisconsin, California, Colorado, Washington, Texas, and Canada. The circle of friends was fairly constant but the place called "home" kept changing. Then eighteen years in a shared house in Seattle, but lots of the time in hotels and on airplanes as I traveled the world to speak about frugality. Then cancer uprooted me from everything, planting me like a seed in that rental on Whidbey. Everywhere I lived until this diet—even Seattle for so many years—felt more like a stage set than settled. That old Willie Nelson song "On the Road Again" used to be my theme song.

Another place I'd claimed as home was "the planet." I was a global citizen. I was part of a highly mobile global community of sustainability pioneers. We met in hotels and at conferences like lovers meet for trysts, sustaining a conversation about "narratives" and "paradigms" and "policy frameworks" and processes and philosophies and levers and systems and who was funding what. We ate at buffets and banquets and in restaurants, and I always came home a few pounds heavier—wherever home was.

It was like I'd hovered over life, one of the privileged few who did not need to land somewhere—or apparently anywhere—to make a go of it. When I was a highflyer, so to speak, I tended to look down on people who stayed put. The term "local yokels" probably went through my mind more than once. "A rolling stone gathers no moss" used to seem an instruction to keep moving. Now it seemed like a formula for never belonging to a place or a people.

With the 10-mile diet I'd landed, and I suspected it wasn't just for a month. I began to understand what being a part of place and community could mean in a different way. Shopping, dancing, walking the trails, strolling in town, I saw Belinda and Koren, Britt and Eric, Sandra and Nina, Tricia, Kent, Pam, and other farmers I knew, like Georgie, Molly and Anna and John Peterson, and Loren and Patty Imes, and on and on. Not only were they becoming part of my life, I was becoming part of theirs.

John Young, a teacher of traditional ways, talks about becoming native to a place. When I'd met him fifteen years earlier he was giving every student an entry-level assignment: Find a "secret spot"—a place in nature near your home that calls you. Visit it daily, rain or shine, chilly or warm, for a year. Notice the life in this small patch— the cycles of the plants, the animal tracks, the changing arc of the sun, the shifting winds. Only then are you ready for the next assignment. He had an "alien test," now called a "tourist test," that asked questions about where you live—about native vegetation, waterways, which direction the storms come from, poisonous plants, and animal tracks. Almost everyone flunked. Almost none of us really lives where we live.

My 10-mile diet was like a secret spot—a place I was, by choice, tethered to. Surprisingly, after so many years of spreading my wings, I found spreading my roots liberating.

The Freedom of Limits

The second thought that came was this: The constraints of this diet had actually freed me from my fierce independence, a brittle shield that did nothing to really allay my fears. I'd bumped into this shield in those six months of contemplation when I had cancer. I'd felt it like a mime feels a wall—invisible but made vivid when contact happens. I was old and wise enough to not try to rip it down or dismiss it as fantasy. I let my life still, let that fluttering self settle down. Now, thanks to the diet, I had settled in. Rather than feeling trapped, I felt held. The ground under me seemed solid. I didn't need to fabricate safety every day by my actions. I just needed to participate.

For years I'd thought, written, and lectured about "liberating limits." How a canvas can free an artist's imagination. How well-made structures (bridges, marriages, cities) actually give people the freedom to move. How values are the chosen limits that allow our lives to deepen rather than dissipate.

My 10-mile diet, with all its constraints, was a perfect case in point. This rootedness was actually freeing me from that background fear. As I looked back over the month from the happy land of toast and almond butter, of chocolate and popcorn, I was able to see how many of what I called problems turned out to be portals into new freedoms. Like all limits, the obstacles interrupted my patterns. To find my way to happiness again, I couldn't go back to blissful ignorance. I went forward, sometimes through thickets of assumptions, to find a truer place to stand and a softer, sweeter sense of freedom.

I reflected on these liberating limits I'd encountered over the past four weeks:

There were unpleasant constraints that turned out to be doorways into a greater love. My flair for drama made me think of myself as a Russian peasant as I packed for that trip to Bellingham. Honest fidelity to my word, though, set me up for an honest realization: love trumps rules. The love poured into purchasing and preparing the food at that conference was a higher value than my strict adherence to a limit I'd set. Only by keeping your word does breaking it in service to a higher truth have any meaning. A more nuanced "rule"—"local everywhere"—came from that surrender. Local isn't consigning oneself to a narrow existence. Rather, "local" is honoring, respecting and supporting the life of the place you are, wherever that is. Without the disrupting limit to my everywhere-eating, I would not have learned these lessons.

There were creative solutions when I couldn't just "go to the store." Missing ingredients snapped me out of my routines and forced me to actually address what I did have with new respect and even gratitude. What I lacked in range I made up for in imagination. Lowly potatoes rose in status in the absence of rice or pasta. I really saw all the possibilities in all the vegetables that grew here. Honey, my only sweetener, became the nectar of the gods, not just an expensive way to widen my girth. Using the ingredients at hand, I figured out how to create a full-spectrum sense of satisfaction—even substitute crunch.

The day I woke up famished and had to make a creamed soup from scratch showed me how little I'd valued the time I'd invested in food preparation. I'd considered it a chore, and discovered it could be self-expression. I'd thought it was a time-suck, but could see it now as self-care. What is more important, really, than conscious cooking and eating? Except for sex, eating is the only time we consciously open ourselves to receive the "not us"—that we allow something from out there into our bodies.

Sure, I could have planned better so that I would have had soup already prepared for my postnap snack, but planning is not my strong suit. I'm inventive to make up for being forgetful and distractible. The restrictions of this diet allowed my inner culinary artist to flourish.

There was a more honest, humble attitude toward the value of my time, with food taking a rightful amount of my attention. The 10-mile diet reduced the importance I give to my persona in the world—writing, speaking, leading. I am not so busy that I can't attend, like everyone else, to the daily acts of harvesting and preparing food. The products of my mind are not more valuable than the products of the earth. I didn't become an obsessive foodie, shucking my other activities. I included relational eating as part of my life.

I matured as an eater from being on the teat of the industrial system to being aware of what it takes to feed me—and all of us. The sticker shock over the five-dollars-a-pound chicken was a blessing—it startled me into respect. My habit of hyperfrugality, ingrained over years, may never change, but now I can see through the plastic on the store-chicken carcass into the life of that bird or one like it. I can see the large industrial chicken houses and compare them to the spacious chicken coop up the hill. Once aware, you can't be fully asleep again. The hidden costs of industrial food are now clear to me, influencing my shopping, cooking, and eating as well as my writing, speaking, and projects.

It now seemed strange how much I had outsourced nourishment to "the experts"—the industrial growers, the packagers, the supermarkets, the cookbooks, the FDA, the USDA, the restaurants. Our industrial system has rendered us as ignorant about where food comes from as we are about how our computers work. Consequently, when we think about nourishment we think about "nutritional content" as listed by "the experts" on the plastic wrappers of foodlike substances. My 10-mile diet had given me an experiential touchstone. I was far less confused and dependent on others to tell me what was right or wrong about the foods I ate.

Looking at how all these challenges—time, lack of the right ingredients, money, planning, inconvenience, hunger—had actually awakened my conscience, my competencies, and my heart to community, I saw how I was finally living that truth of "liberating limits."

Shifting from Lone Ranger freedom, I saw that community is also freeing. I used to quip, "Everyone wants community. Unfortunately, that involves other people." Our habits of hyperindividualism have isolated us, making us more insecure rather than more secure, more fragile rather than stronger—but what a hard habit to break! The 10-mile diet, a hard nut to crack, actually cracked me open.

Food Rules

What rules—chosen constraints—might keep me on this path? How might I be faithful to what I now know, not like a convert to a cause but like a quiet daily attentiveness? By now, nearly at the end of the month, it was natural to think out loud about this by blogging. I wrote:

Here are my 10-mile derived truths—which have rules associated with them. Rules that I will surely break but that will be there for me from this day forward.

1. All food comes from somewhere. I want to find out where so I can in a way thank those that feed me, reward good practices and protect the livelihood of small to mid-sized farmers (sounds funny, I mean the land not the people). This could be a daunting but fascinating task. Eating local solves that issue so . . .

Rule: I will purchase as much as possible direct from the producer.

2. Food is love. Producing it. Cooking it. Eating it so that your body may be nourished. Death as an animal or vegetable and rebirth as us, living one more day. Our own death, if we don't rest and rot forever in stainless steel boxes, feeds life. This doesn't imply we must slather eating with unctuous sanctity, but that we can make a good faith effort to honor the life sacrificed that we may eat. In the community where I lived for 35 years we said grace before every meal. "Rub dub thanks for the grub. Bless this food to our use and our lives to your service. Thank you." The pausing and holding hands bound us together at the end of busy dispersed days, slowed us down to the speed of savoring. Food is social. I will simply eat more with others, cook more for others, eat out with others. I will glory in my ability to feed people, to take from my stores and make a feast (if only fried rice) for friends.

Rule: I will say grace, eat slowly and savor my food, and with others as often as possible in my solo, willful and busy life. I will cook for others as much as possible. From scratch.

3. I am my food system, not apart from it picking and choosing but part of it, giving and receiving. This is a shift from food being out there in a supermarket where we select this over that. Once you see yourself as woven into a food system, not just a shopper in a market where the system is hidden from view, more than what goes into your mouth transforms you.

Rule: I will allow my life as an eater to make me aware of the web of life that supports me, and all of us. I can use a phrase as simple as "food system" to remember.

4. *Food is political, there's no way around it.* From raw milk being illegal to other distorting government policies that make packaged food cheaper than real food. From school lunches of pizza and purple milk to the ever growing number of hungry in our midst.

Rule: I will inform myself about the food system, the regulations and laws and customs that give us both obesity and starvation. I will vote about it. I will write about it. I will donate.

5. *Food is complex.* The way we live is shaped around the food we eat even when eating is done in cars, in cities, far from the source. Agriculture, as we all know from our history and geography lessons, permitted humans to settle in one place which permitted social stratification in cities, money, specialization, slavery—you name it, taming grains and animals gave it to you. Humans now occupy almost all niches where energy (food) is available for the picking or planting. Civilization itself has marched across the face of the earth—as Bonaparte said of armies—on its stomach.

Breakthroughs in food technologies—the Green Revolution, selective breeding, genetic modification, industrial agriculture, even the Farm Bill—solve the problems of starvation while feeding the problems of diminishing productivity and a population that now is so large it seems we can't all be fed.

Food is complex because of this history and its unintended consequences. The food problem is the overshoot problem which is the annual increase of births over deaths problem, and if you want a hot potato try talking about that! I am dedicated to the work of "learning to live well together within the means of the earth." No amount of "Eat your peas, think of the starving children in China/Korea/Bangladesh/Pakistan/Africa" can solve our malnourishment and maldistribution problems. They are systemic. Hunger, I fear, is going to creep into lives that thought they were secure. And when we are hungry we are cranky. So add war to the list.

Rule: I can nudge the system in the right direction with my choices and I intend to. I will support local sustainable agriculture everywhere.

6. *Food is highly emotionally charged.* People have pride and shame, fear and

longing around weight, size, diet du jour, longevity, inability to feed the family, diet-related illness. And I am people. I am a lifelong "diet-er"—and even if I were thin as a rail I'd still somehow have an eating disorder since I look at food as a threat or reward, as comfort or sport, as right and wrong—and myself as good or bad depending on which system I'm beating myself up with now.

Rule: When I find myself judging myself, others or others' judgments of me I will step back, get grounded and let go.

7. Food is great. Tasty, tangy, creamy, yummy, oily, colorful, salty, biting, sweet, juicy, spicy, crunchy, crisp, meaty, fishy, slithery, chewy, nutty, hot, refreshing, subtle. Lord strike me dumb at least (or dumber) if I don't fully savor every bite of that miracle called food.

Rule: I will enjoy the sensual, delicious act of eating.

8. Food is fun. It's always there to select and cook and eat, to think about, to learn about, to write about and especially enjoy. It shouldn't be stuck between "more important things," like a gas station or pit stop for the body. 10-mile eating isn't a new food system. A new set of imperatives. I have stumbled into a new relationship with food. I can offer others this way of engaging with food—which may result in more justice, health, appropriate weight, sustainability and fun. What do you think?

Rule: Continue to write about, think about, research, advocate for—and eat—food. Bon Appetit.

La-De-Da

Then a most sobering thought overtook my wandering mind.

This experiment was not going to be over on October 1. I'd committed to the 50/50 February experiment. Me and my big mouth.

As this reality sank in I realized that I needed to start thinking ahead. Where was my food for the winter months going to come from? The only thing that survives in my garden over the winter is kale. I've seen it with an inch of snow on top. I've seen it glazed with ice like some plastic Christmas tree. It still survives. But no woman can live on kale alone.

Welcome to the reality of fall for most of human history. Not fall as the time to start a seasonal marathon of pigging out on trick-or-treat loot or turkey and stuffing. (And by the way, pigs do not pig out. Few animals do, except when they hang out with us.)

No, traditionally fall meant the seasonal race to preserve all that great food before it rotted. It was its own marathon of canning, drying, freezing, digging, picking, burying (potatoes and turnips can be buried in dry sand), and even planting for early spring. Fall meant hours of blanching and pickling and chopping and scalding. Fall meant falling into bed exhausted having put up green beans, green tomato chutney, tomatoes, zucchini puree for soups, squash puree for pies, applesauce, and chicken.

Yes, I said chicken. My ultra-energy-efficient freezer accomplishes this energy savings partly because it is so small—too small for a whole month's worth of meat, fruit, and vegetables. It was made in Europe, where many people still eat in moderation, still shop daily, wheeling their rickety wire carts to the butcher, fishmonger, and green grocer to see what is fresh and appealing. We in America, on the other hand, treat our fridges like storage lockers—stuffing them with items we may never use. As George Carlin once said, "Leftovers make you feel good twice. First, when you put it away, you feel thrifty and intelligent: 'I'm saving food!' Then a month later when blue hair is growing out of the ham and you throw it away, you feel really intelligent: 'I'm saving my life!'" So, if I wanted meat and veggies in February, I needed to do at least a bit of canning.

How could I do that on the cheap? Belinda had some tough old hens that no longer laid enough eggs to pay for their feed. (Life is harsh on the farm.) She cheerfully sold me three—plucked, gutted, and frozen—for half the price I'd pay for a tender young fryer, and threw in the canning directions for free. "Just stick the pieces whole in the jar. Don't bother to bone them. They'll can just fine."

In the past I'd butchered everything from a pig to a coon, not to mention chickens, rabbits, and our ornery rooster named Holy Fu*k. I was sure once I'd sharpened my knife I'd whip through those birds, putting the meat in jars and making the bones into broth.

Not.

Those old birds really knew how to hang together—thighs to legs, wings to backs, breasts to thighs. Picture me hunched over my cutting board, arms flapping like chicken wings, hacking and pounding while I chewed on my pride so I could swallow it. I ended up boiling the whole carcasses enough to soften the ligaments. I then boned them, boiled six canning jars, packed them with meat, filled them to a half inch of the top with broth, wiped the sealing edges carefully, popped the sterilized lids on carefully, screwed on the retaining rings, put them in my forty-year-old canner, added several inches of water, tightened the lug nuts, put it on a burner set to high, vented the steam, put the fifteen pounds of pressure weight on, waited for the jiggle, turned down the heat, and pressure-canned those suckers for ninety minutes. All for six pints of chicken.

Yet there can be a great deal of satisfaction and even pleasure in doing the work associated with feeding our families. Looking at a well-stocked pantry or freezer, knowing where that food came from and where it will go, you can feel a real sense of accomplishment and—dare I say it—love. Food from your hands and heart will feed people you care about. The last time I knew I would not starve because I had stored food was that winter nearly forty years earlier in Rhinelander when we stored packages labeled Sue (Piggy Sue), Jane (Jane Doe the deer), Dr. Buck (the deer), and Stew (the steer) in our neighbor's freezer. We just don't have to think that way anymore, such a recent development in human history. I don't presume we'll need to go to my extremes anytime soon, but there is no better way to develop a truly visceral relationship with food than to store in September what you will eat in the winter.

What Else Is on the 50/50 February Shopping List?

Six pints of chicken, though, would not go very far.

Fortunately, my 10-mile month made this 50/50 constraint feel like taking off a tight girdle and sprawling on the sofa. I could go farther to find food. I could also go beyond even those fifty miles to eat what I damn well pleased, in moderation.

It was simple to check my supplies at home and my known suppliers to verify I'd be covered.

Milk: I had my regular suppliers.

Meat: still had plenty of the Long Family beef, plus a few Tobey chickens.

Exotics: check. Double check, in fact, because I had to do only 50 percent.

But for the rest . . . I needed to do some serious thinking.

It was time to start enlarging my pool of food suppliers and range of foods. So when I was at the market that Saturday I talked to Georgie Smith, a fourth-generation farmer from Ebey's Prairie, a mere twenty-five miles north. She shares a booth at the market with Mike Nichols, who started as a farmer and is now developing a local food delivery service, picking up from island growers—and beyond—and delivering to customers' doorsteps.

Mike may be too young to be a true curmudgeon, but he's a curmudgeon-in-training—wiry and compact with rugged good looks, a wry sense of humor, and strong opinions. As a grower he was well aware of a missing link between small producers and their customers. Every one of them needed a truck and time to bring their product to market. He decided to fill this gap with Whidbey Green Goods, buying surplus from gardeners and farmers and delivering custom orders to his clients each week. By cultivating this very local ground, Mike is actually generating more island production as people realize they can put in one more row of beans and fund a year of movies. He says of his endeavor, "One rung up the food ladder from 'home garden' is a food web of small growers and producers that are of a size where they give a damn about what they grow and produce to put on your table! Whidbey Green Goods is your link to that Very Local food web. . . . WGG's primary mission is to move this Very Local bounty into Very Local kitchens."

One of his biggest suppliers is the very Georgie Smith who shares his stand.

Georgie is a big, bosomy, ruddy-cheeked no-nonsense woman who decided to put five-plus acres of her family's rich bottomland in production when the economy sank and took her ten-year job as a marketing director at a small import company with it. Her farmer's capacity to improvise solutions and her dad's ability to cobble together anything needed from old parts has made her business flourish. She grows many kinds of vegetables but specializes in heirloom dried beans and a variety of potatoes and onions. I strapped a ten-pound bag of potatoes to my bike carrier, added some onions and a bag of beans to the saddlebag, paid gladly, sauntered over to the Island Apiaries booth for my February honey, and then pedaled home. Even with all that weight on board, I got up the hill and into the garage. When I hung my net bag of potatoes on the unused garage door tracks, I felt a bit like a hunter who'd arrived with a dressed deer strapped onto my Land Rover's roof.

Later in the fall I called Mike for a home delivery of several squash, which I proudly displayed above my kitchen cupboards as if they were Grandma's fine crockery. I had several of my own mystery squash up there as well. They had grown to basketball size on sprawling squash plants from seed someone had given me. If I wondered how I'd fare in the winter, I just needed to look up there, calculating two meals a squash, and look at the bag of potatoes, calculating about twenty meals per bag, and open my onion drawer or check my garlic bowl or, of course, look at my jars of Belinda's chicken. I could open my freezer to check on the two local chickens resting silently beside a beef roast and some liver. My stores were limited, yes, but they were THERE.

Then I discovered Georgie's neighbors on Ebey's Prairie, grain growers Georgina Silby and Lauren Hubbard. Grains meant—if I would grind them—everything bread-y and pasta-y and cracker-y. Grains, I now realized, having lived largely on vegetables, meant stick-to-your-ribs, solid-in-the-belly food. I understood for the first time the elegance of grains, a calorie-dense, nutrient-rich, easily stored and transported food, and, in fact, the foundation of civilization. I was ready to stock up.

Georgina Silby sold me two pounds of Tibetan purple barley—hand-packed in recyclable brown paper bags. The price per pound was high, but the integrity in that grain was priceless. Even when I see her in jeans and a threadbare shirt, her long neck, porcelain skin, and beauty make me think of lawns and manors, not fields and manure. Georgina grew up in Wales and landed on Whidbey because her godparents live here. Her commitment to grain farming has many roots, so to speak. She's steeped in earth-based spirituality. She was a leader in the anti-GMO movement in the UK. She believes—and teaches—that food is medicine, and she has a broad knowledge of herbalism. You can almost taste all this in her barley. A small bowl is filling and delicious and something else intangible: a felt sense of nourishment.

Lauren Hubbard, who also grows grains on the Prairie, graduated magna cum laude from Washington State University, where she had been an award-winning communications, women's studies, and soil science major, but instead of making a career in those professional fields, her path led her back to the fields on Ebey's Prairie with her husband, Clark Bishop. The Bishops are one of the key farming families on Ebey's Prairie, and by marrying Clark Bishop (the sixth generation on their land), Lauren married into a future of agriculture . . . if they as a couple wanted that life. A stint in the peace corps in Moldova working with farmers in the former breadbasket of the Soviet Union, where the fall of communism fragmented the agricultural system, convinced them that they did. They saw the farming system spin into a nosedive, with too little land and too many regulations wringing the life out of the people. Lauren and Clark realized they were privileged to be able to farm his family's land and surprised themselves by returning to the prairie—grounded in science and ready to muck in the dirt as farmers. So here they are, bridging from the farming style of Clark's parents to the consumer preferences for local organic food. I bought ten pounds of her emmer (a precursor of wheat), intending to both grind it for breads (with my Good Cheer thrift-store find, a new-in-the-box, bolted-to-the-counter hand grinder) and eat it in pilafs.

With just barley, emmer, and beans added to my stores of squash, chicken, beef, potatoes, and onions, I had enough basic food to fulfill my 50 percent commitment.

I learned some tricks for cooking these grains and beans from scratch. I soak the beans for at least thirty-six hours, changing the water a couple of times (like when I notice). That cuts the cooking time by 60 percent and also sprouts the beans, which increases the nutrition. I then rinse the beans, cover with water in a pressure cooker, bring them to a boil, drain, rinse, and then cover with water again, pressure-cook the beans for five minutes at five pounds of pressure with a piece of kombu seaweed, which takes the toot right out of them. I soak the grains too for a day or two. Sprouted grains are more digestible and nutritious. Same really quick, slick pressure-cooking, though a little longer. They are so nutritious that half a cup fills me up.

I checked with Tricia about what she could provide in the winter. She really didn't have eggs to spare, but on a tour of The Goose Community Grocer I found John Whitney stocking local Skymeadow eggs. He gave me an earful about eggs, and by now I was absolutely fascinated by all things edible and local, so we lingered for half an hour between the dairy case and bulk food aisles as I grilled him. To sell at the Goose he had to provide a bottomless supply of eggs a day, washed and packed according to the USDA Egg Products Inspection Act and the Washington Wholesome Eggs and Egg Products Act. His operation must be licensed and insured and records must be kept in detail for two years. I haven't met a small businessman who really likes regulations and licensing, but John had run the gauntlet and made it work. He and his wife, Else, had ramped up their egg production to be able to meet the standards of quality and quantity that the supermarkets require.

"Why not organic?" I asked.

"The annual inspection alone is one thousand dollars. I can't afford it. And the record keeping is way too much for us. Our eggs are as good as organic, but we just can't make the certification work." I heard this story again and again. To the dismay of many of the pioneers whose blood, sweat, and tears enshrined the National Organic Standards in the USDA, small-scale local producers with loyal customers are not investing time and energy to get certified. Local meat and dairy on a rural island like Whidbey may well not be *certified* organic—and may not even be licensed. Another lesson is the dual system for trusting our food: I need to either look in the eye of the farmer or look at a label that is backed by rigorous requirements, testing, and verifications.

I was grateful that John and Else had jumped through all the hoops necessary to get local eggs into my local market. I'd have eggs in February! It's not easy for small farmers to provide sufficiently plentiful and reliable products to merit shelf or bin space in the supermarkets.

Several weeks later, after the 10-mile pressure had simmered down, I met John and Else at the farmers' market. They'd been there all along, but my need for eggs hadn't been great enough for their presence to make much of a difference. Else and I chatted egg business knowledgeably, me drawing on that detailed conversation at the Goose, and by the end she shared a little secret. The bigger eggs wouldn't fit in the egg cartons without cracking, so she sold them from a little fridge on her porch for a tad less. More for less. That sounded like just my cup of tea. Once I had her address, I had my egg supply for the winter and beyond sewn up.

There would be no cheese from Nina, though, and Vicky Brown's girls would be nursing their kids in the late winter, but I could get Mt. Townsend Creamery cheese across the water on the Kitsap Peninsula, or default to anywhere cheese and count it in my 50 percent nonlocal. Likewise other essential exotics, like nuts and nut butters.

There! I was prepared for a fairly peasant-y February. Then, as D-Day (diet day) approached, I met Jess Dowdell.

Jess is a wiry, redheaded chef who worked at the time at Ca'buni, a café in the large foyer of a warehouse that is primarily a coffee roaster and occasionally a performance space for live jazz, blues, and comedy. It's in the woods, down a bumpy, only partially paved road, but that doesn't stop a loyal following from eating, drinking, and being entertained there. Ca'buni means casa (home) in the boonies.

Jess is committed to serving a local menu. She is our local version of Alice Waters of Chez Panisse in Berkeley and Judy Wicks of the White Dog Café in Philadelphia, women chefs who have pioneered the growing trend of restaurateurs' becoming agents of change in local food systems. Many chefs, responding to a demand for local food on the menu, will buy whatever is fresh from farmers through the back kitchen door, but these women also drive the market. They are quantity buyers, and when they add a dish to their menu they become volume buyers.

Jess explained this over Numi tea one day at Ca'buni. After a rapid-fire critique of the industrial food system using a tone reserved for really rotten movies, she revealed her suppliers and strategies for serving a local menu every day to a steady stream of customers.

She gets her pork from the original heritage breed pig at Chia, a small family-owned and -operated farm in Clinton, the first unincorporated town on the island, right off the ferry. Her beef comes from 3 Sisters Cattle Company at the north end. The three sisters are the daughters of Ron and Shelly Muzzall, fourth-generation farmers on Whidbey Island, who built the business of supplying quality USDA-approved beef—grass-fed grain-finished steers that pasture in the summer and eat grain grown right on the farm over the winter.

Jess gets her chickens from Skagit Valley just north and east over the Deception Pass Bridge.

Her vegetables come from Quail's Run Farm in Clinton, where Loren and Patty Imes custom-grow for Jess's annual menu. She gives them a list of seeds they need to buy, pays them as if they were a CSA (which they are, but for a restaurant, not a family), and gets a steady supply of vegetables from spring through fall.

This is a boon to Loren and Patti, but still does not cover expenses for a family of four. Like most small farmers, they need a second income to make ends meet. Loren does Web design to support the family, just like Britt and Eric need her income from nonprofit work to survive. Tricia's farm income is only one small part of her and Kent's household income, with his job as a teacher being the main source of green stuff.

Sprouts come from Ferry View Farms in Clinton. Chanterelles come from the forests and the oysters from beds right in Holmes Harbor.

Jess gets her heirloom pumpkins from another grower and her eggs from my very own supplier, Skymeadow.

What tomatoes Loren and Patty can't provide year-round Jess gets from small organic family farms in Mexico.

She visits as many of her farmers as she can at least twice a year. She wants to see the cows and visit the chickens and know the families and be sure everything—from land to animals to vegetables to children—is well loved.

"It's not just where your food comes from. It's who grows it, and how sustainable their lives are."

The coffee, of course, is Mukilteo, roasted right in the warehouse. Owner Gary's ethic mirrors Jess's. He buys direct from farmers around the world and likes to go to the farms and meet the growers.

For tea Jess picked Numi, a fair trade company, which we were drinking as we chatted.

And some of what doesn't grow on the island grows in our fifty-mile food shed. She loves shopping at the Ballard farmers' market in Seattle and clubbing afterward—and it helps that provisioning for Ca'buni requires trips to the mainland.

"Come with me," she offered.

"For sure," I said, very keen to expand my repertoire for February.

Ballard is the old Scandihoovian ("Scandinavian" in Ballardese) fishing neighborhood of Seattle, now filling with standard jeans-and-fleece young families types, topped with ever more hip coffee shops and bars. This farmers' market, like many other flourishing ones, is a feast for the senses. There are ethnic-food stalls, baked goods, foraged fungi from the forests, music, and handcrafted gifts. Jess directed me to her favorite, Nash's from Sequim on the Olympic Peninsula. They had a large stand with tables heaped high with greens, cabbages and Brussels sprouts, roots, grains, squash, and potatoes. Not everyone pounces on parsnip, but I have relished them roasted and mashed ever since discovering them wild in cow pastures in Rhinelander—and stocked up. I got some greens, cabbage, and Brussels sprouts (another delicacy when roasted), all the while chatting with the young woman farmer in a watch cap and frayed hoodie about my 10-mile diet and upcoming 50-mile experiment. She liked my story and threw in a free bag of rye berries with my order. From another stand I bought two more five-dollars-a-pound chickens for the freezer.

When I was a global eater, ten miles was a struggle. Compared to that, fifty miles—with roots and squash and flour and barley and beans and winter greens—was heaven.

I was stocked and stoked, ready for February 1. I could have as many exotics as I wanted as long as 50 percent of my nourishment stayed within a few hours' drive. Ready. Set. Eat.

WHY I FARM

I asked my farmers these questions—and below are their answers.

- Why do you farm?
- What makes it rewarding despite all the difficulties?
- What makes it tough?
- Do you have a philosophy of farming?
- What do you want eaters to know that they might not?

GEORGIE SMITH, A WRITER HERSELF, HAD A LOT TO SAY.
HERE ARE EXCERPTS:

"[I farm] because I can't not farm. Farmers don't become farmers to make a million dollars. They do it because that is who they are. Then the struggle is how to match up who you are with how to make it financially viable."

"The reward is seeing a crop brought to harvest at the end of the day, when you are body-tired but mind-satisfied by the tasks accomplished. [And it is] not nebulous in its importance (how important TRULY is that new Gap shirt? or the latest iPhone?). It is food. It sustains and nourishes and provides life."

"[It's hard because] food has been taken for granted for a long time in this country. Often when I deliver my weekly orders I stop by to buy office supplies. It is not common for me to spend easily the same amount in buying a bit of paper, ink, a few pens, maybe some staples, as I have just made in one or two of my deliveries. That always seems skewed to me. We have devalued the price of the things we need most to survive on a daily basis yet overvalued many of the things we can live without."

"[Not only that but] farmers are the ultimate gamblers. Sure, there are crop insurance plans you can sign up for, but for farmers like me, working on a smaller, very diversified level with many crops, I don't quality for insurance. So every year I take a risk that the garlic won't rot due to an unseasonably wet spring, the potatoes won't succumb to blight due to a warm and wet summer, the dry beans will get enough heat to grow and mature before the fall rains hit."

"[My] philosophy is 'sustainability.' And by that I mean not only farming using sustainable practices to nurture the land but the financial sustainability of what I do, and the emotional and physical sustainability of

what I do. If I cannot find a way to farm that provides enough financial reward while allowing me enough time to relax and recover and enjoy my family, then it doesn't matter how great of an 'environmentally sustainable' farmer I am, I can't financially and emotionally/physically sustain it."

"I don't think that eaters/consumers know how much work goes into almost every crop, not to mention how often crops fail. People will often say to me, 'Wow, Georgie . . . you have a really green thumb.' My response is, Not really, I just plant A LOT."

PAM MITCHELL IS QUITE THE OPPOSITE—
A WOMAN OF FEW WORDS. SHE SAID:

"Mother Earth is the greatest partner I've ever had. She provides me an excellent education in mutually supportive collaboration. I'm astonished by Her generosity, grateful for Her wisdom, and humbled by Her patience. She is truly the love of my life."

GEORGINA SILBY, WHO GROWS BIODYNAMIC GRAINS,
BROUGHT HER SPIRITUAL VALUES TO HER ANSWERS

"I farm primarily to be intimately connected with the dance of life, to build soil, and to produce high-quality food for the well-being of humans. As an aspiring biodynamic farmer, I am learning how to mediate the forces above and below. Plants are some of my greatest teachers, and so to work with them is very satisfying. I also love to be outside and engaged in creative production."

"Being connected to the alchemy of farming is deeply nourishing, and learning about how life really works is humbling. Observing the soil's transformation is very inspiring, especially when it is increasing in its biological activity and tilth. It's also very rewarding to eat good food that I was personally involved in creating."

"My economic challenges are similar to other start-up businesses. There is no living wage for me at this time. I am still marketing and getting established as a local producer. In addition to the weather factor, I am dependent on other farmers for their equipment, and that can be very hard, like the time my crops were perfectly ripe and ready for harvest but it was Labor Day weekend and I could not get anyone to bring their combine over to my fields. Then it rained and the crops were compromised."

"My farming philosophy is quite influenced by old earth-based traditions of various agrarian societies. . . . I look at the land as a living organism, and consider how to keep it in a regenerative state. I choose not to plow, and prioritize building the soil. This is like the immune system; if the soil is balanced and healthy, the crops will generally respond accordingly. I pay attention to cosmic influences also; the sun is not the only heavenly body that determines outcomes in the field. Observation and listening are perhaps the most important practices for me; paying careful attention to as much as possible, and then being appropriately guided. Feedback from the plants is crucial, and not just the ones I intentionally planted; the weeds are great indicators also. And then there are other farmers; their observations and shared insights are priceless, and help me tremendously."

"[I want eaters to know] that farm food is stardust transformed by the elementals. That the intention of the farmer deeply affects the quality of the food. Some people know why local honey is important, but that principle applies to eating any local food. It is healthier since the plants and animals from your area are better adapted to your local conditions (same air, same rain . . .) and so offer humans specific support in subtle but significant ways."

FINALLY, ANNIE JESPERSON:

I met Annie when she was a student at the Greenbank Farm Training Center. She is now, with her partner, Nathaniel, farming on Molly and John Peterson's land. She says:

"I farm because farming allows me to use my entire being—my body, mind, and soul—to work toward the health of my community. Through this beautiful, challenging work I get to be a philosopher and a scientist, an educator and an activist, a dreamer and a doer—employing all my faculties to nurture crops, build soil, and promote well-being for the people within my reach. My heroes are small-scale farmers, whose lives are guided not by the allure of immense profits but by love of hard work, of people, and of land. I want to someday emanate the wisdom and love that they've acquired through years of embracing this tough, dirty, and all-important work. Through farming, I have the chance to use my creativity, my strength, and my heart every day to do something that I find incredibly rewarding. This is why I farm."

Now It's Your Turn

If you live with others but don't eat together, establish a once-a-day or twice-a-week or even just once-a-week ritual of dining together. Say grace. Have a conversation where everyone has a chance to speak. Enjoy the stories of each person's day or week.

Yes! magazine collected some graces from around the world.[1]

Buddhist

This food is the gift
of the whole universe.
Each morsel is a sacrifice of life,
May I be worthy to receive it.
May the energy in this food
Give me the strength
To transform my unwholesome qualities
Into wholesome ones.
I am grateful for this food.
May I realize the Path of Awakening,
For the sake of all beings.

Ashanti (Ghana)

Earth, when I am about to die
I lean upon you.
Earth, while I am alive
I depend upon you.

Christian Children's Prayer

Thank you God for the world so sweet,
Thank you God for the food we eat.
Thank you God for the birds that sing,
Thank you God for everything.

Hindu (India)

Before grasping this grain,
let us consider in our minds
the reasons why
we should care for and safeguard this body.
This is my prayer, oh God:
May I be forever devoted at your feet,
offering body, mind, and wealth
to the service of truth in the world.

Mother Teresa, Catholic (Calcutta, India)

Make us worthy, Lord,
To serve those people
Throughout the world who live and die
In poverty and hunger.
Give them, through our hands
This day their daily bread,
And by our understanding love,
Give peace and joy.

Sioux

I'm an Indian.
I think about the common things like this pot.
The bubbling water comes from the rain cloud.
It represents the sky.
The fire comes from the sun,
Which warms us all, men, animals, trees.
The meat stands for the four-legged creatures,
Our animal brothers,
Who gave themselves so that we should live.
The steam is living breath.
It was water, now it goes up to the sky,
Becomes a cloud again.
These things are sacred.
Looking at that pot full of good soup,
I am thinking how, in this simple manner,
The Great Spirit takes care of me.

Jewish

Praised are You, our God, Ruler of the universe, who in goodness, with grace,
kindness, and mercy, feeds the entire world. He provides bread for all creatures,
for His kindness is never-ending. And because of His magnificent greatness we
have never wanted for food, nor will we ever want for food, to the end of time.

For His great name, because He is God who feeds and provides for all, and
who does good to all by preparing food for all of His creatures whom He created:
Praised are You, God, who feeds all.

Try These Recipes

Georgie Smith's signature crop is Rockwell beans, a traditional Whidbey dry bean, so here's the right place to get her grandma Smith's recipe. And since I found some parsnips for my 50-mile diet at Nash's, I'm including Jess Dowdell's recipe for Parsnip and Aged Sheep Cheese Gratin.

Georgie's Grandma Smith's Rockwell Baked Beans

2–3 cups Rockwell beans (each cup is 2–3 servings)
1 medium-to-large onion, chopped
4–5 large garlic cloves, chopped into large chunks
1 small package cured salt pork, cut into 1-inch chunks
½–1 cup brown sugar
¼–½ cup dry mustard
Salt and pepper to taste

Soak the beans overnight.
Preheat the oven to 325°F.
Place the beans in a 2-quart oven-safe casserole dish with a lid. Add the onion, garlic, salt pork, and half of the brown sugar and dry mustard. Add enough water to cover the beans by about double their depth. Put the lid on and place in the preheated oven. Bake for 3 to 4 hours. Check every 30 minutes, stirring and adding water if the beans start to dry out. When the beans are soft and creamy, add more brown sugar, dry mustard, salt, and pepper as desired. Take the lid off and cook an additional 15 minutes to caramelize the top and cook off any excess water.

Jess's Parsnip and Aged Sheep Cheese Gratin

8–10 parsnips, sliced about ⅛ inch thick
3 cups goat's milk
1 cup cow's heavy cream
1 cup vegetable stock
4 teaspoons whole-grain mustard
1 cup grated aged sheep cheese (I love Glendale Shepherd's Brebis cheese)

Parboil the parsnips for 3 minutes, then rinse in cold water to cool them down quickly.

In a bowl combine the goat's milk, cow's cream, vegetable stock, mustard, and ½ cup of the grated cheese.

Oil the bottom of a 13-inch roasting pan. Lay down one layer of the parsnips, drizzle with the milk mixture, and repeat this process until you have finished all the parsnips. Cover with the remaining milk mixture, then cover the pan with foil and bake at 350°F for an hour. Top the gratin with the rest of the cheese and bake uncovered for 10 more minutes, just to melt the cheese.

You can add so much to this one little dish—grated carrots, mustard greens, garlic, leeks, onions, and more or less cream. This is fun, so just go crazy with whatever is in season and local.

CHAPTER EIGHT

Relational Eating

Relational eating was not why I began the 10-mile diet. My reasons were partly sassy (sustainability as extreme sport) and partly serious (in the face of the triple crisis, relocalization was the only thing that made sense).

Relational eating, though, is where I landed. Literally. I came home to eat.

Relational eating crept up on me through my September days of boxes on the counter from Tricia and happening upon the Longs' meat sale on the way to Britt and Eric's wedding. It came through my conversations over contraband milk with Belinda and over a gifted goat leg with Sandra. It shone through Chris Wolfe's eyes as she recounted the local origins of every morsel on our plates in Bellingham, and it came up through my feet in my backyard.

After my first postchallenge bite of toast, still slathered with my hand-churned butter, I walked back into the land of anywhere eating—the land of hard cheeses and nuts and chocolate—but I brought my 10-mile foods along with me. They were all keepers. Anywhere eating was no longer the reward for being a good girl for a month. It had become how I sourced foods I couldn't find closer to home.

I looked at my experience of local food and recognized that it had indeed shifted from commerce to relationship, from weighing and measuring to immeasurables like belonging and love. It wasn't about better "food." It was about a better relationship with food and all the hands that feed me: the farmers and fields that had nourished me, the daily interactions that now were part of my "sustenance." My food, like my grocery store and my movie theater, now had a name tag rather than a bar code.

Throughout October I kept on eating Skymeadow eggs and drinking Elsie's milk. I was still picking greens from my garden and had signed up for Molly Peterson's season-extender CSA, so root crops and greens and squash were still pouring into my fridge and pantry every week. My freezer was still full of Long Family beef and some Tobey chicken. I'd stocked up on Georgie Smith's beans and Georgina Silby's biodynamically grown barley. I had my own and Georgie's and Tricia's squash on top of my cupboards, displayed like family heirlooms. I had jars of applesauce gleaned from a number of island trees, and jars of Belinda's tough old birds. Fifty percent within fifty miles in February now seemed like a piece of cake . . . which I might also have since I had Lauren's emmer and honey from Island Apiaries.

See what I mean? My food had gone from industrial to intimate— but there were even more transformations beyond the provenance of my food:

- My relationship with my body shifted. Instead of it being a possession I judged, adorned, displayed, fed, and used as I liked, I saw it now as a living, breathing part of a living landscape. When I take three deep breaths to start meditation, I am not just relaxing my body, I am filling my lungs and belly with "here." Here receives my feet as I walk.

- My relationship with food has shifted. Instead of yo-yoing between gluttony and "dieting," I actually enjoy food. It's the relational part that made the difference. I get intimacy and nourishment now, not just flavor and . . . OMG, calories. The word *diet* has come to mean what one eats "here"—just as people have done for centuries.

- My relationship with my community has shifted. I had no idea how much of a visitor I was, even owning a home. I had no real stake in the place—in the people or nature. Through local eating, I actually came home.

• My relationship with cooking has shifted. From someone with an adequate repertoire of dishes I liked, I have become a cook with the growing ability to "feel" what I might do with this root or leaf or fruit or muscle right in front of me, and how I might honor its qualities by cooking it well.

• My relationship with entitlement even changed. The unconscious privilege afforded me by my class, education, and experiences has switched to a humble awareness that whoever my ego imagines I am, the reality is that I live by the grace of what lives around me.

• Finally, my relationship with activism changed. I'm no longer fueled by an underlying terror at what my species is making of this world and am motivated now by a real sense that our lives can truly be a blessing for the earth.

All of this is bundled in the term "relational eating."

The Web of Eating

Relational eating encompasses the whole shift from eating as a private affair from a vast continuous smorgasbord heaped high by the largely invisible industrial food system to eating in a living food system where food is precious because I know the farmers, the farms, the farm animals, the fruits and foraging spots, and the vicissitudes of the seasons. Relational eating involves my heart and soul, not just my mouth, because I now live somewhere, not just anywhere.

When I was a kid I was presented with a puzzling question: "Do you eat to live or live to eat?" I didn't know the answer, but wanted to get it right. If I eat to live, that denies all the pleasures of eating—the tastes of oatmeal for breakfast and chopped meat sandwiches for lunch and roast beef for supper, the warmth of dinner with my family, Almond Joys. But if I live to eat, that means I'm all about food, and that could lead to finger pointing to my size. I was stumped.

I couldn't see—until my 10-mile diet—that the question presumed I had no relationship with the food I eat—that I was an eater without any context. Relational eating says we never eat out of context. We always eat food from somewhere, always make food choices in the context of history and culture, climate and geography. Even if we are blissfully or woefully unaware of the fact, food doesn't just appear in a replicator on the *Starship Enterprise*.

I now want to go back to the kids who stumped me and say with a bit of my own gotcha, "You've got it wrong. I love what I eat. And who grows it. I love to feed people. I love being alive. Here."

No one lives outside the web of life. Plants and animals gave their lives so that we might live. Farmers or hunters or ranchers or foragers harvested this food for us, digging or picking or slaughtering or felling. The food may have traveled only a few feet or halfway around the world, with one hand or many hands touching or lifting or sifting or sorting or wrapping or washing it. We chew and savor and soon enough this life is in us, nourishing our bodies, feeding the billions of bacteria in our digestive tract.

Relational eating heals this illusion of isolation from "the hands that feed us" and shows us how deeply we belong to one another.

Belonging

I remember my first experience of belonging here on Whidbey. I was fairly reclusive in the months after I moved into my over-the-garage apartment in March 2005, where I continued my recovery from cancer as I relished that return to anonymity after years in the public eye. Summer came and went, bringing the usual tide of tourists that subsides after Labor Day. In October, the cashier at the Star Store said, as she rang me up, "You left your gloves here last time." I was enough a part of here that when she found my gloves, she knew they were mine and held on to them until I came in again.

Growing up I learned that belonging meant beholden. It meant others owned me and had control over my choices. Here, though, I've slowly relaxed and learned that belonging doesn't have to mean kowtowing. It doesn't mean conformity, putting on a uniform, and getting stripped of your personality, like belonging to the army. It means that even though we may be as different as a hand and a heart, we belong to the same body—in fact, we help determine what that body is. There are limits to appropriate behavior, but they apply to all of us. If we are here and we don't willfully make life tough for one another, we belong.

This is the Goldilocks quality to belonging. To belong you can't be too big for your britches or too much of a shrinking violet. You need to be "just right." In anonymous eating, you can gorge or starve, and who cares? You can buy anything you want, and who's watching, especially if you buy your food at a drive-through? You can be bombastic or a wimp, and you're just part of the daily din of life. Not on my island, or in almost any close-knit community. The more woven into this place I've become, the more I see that my choices matter, for better or worse. I see how others feed my life, and how I also feed them.

Although I now belong here, this community doesn't own me. I'm free to close my door, to live as I wish, to come and go and be a "no-account," not accountable to anyone I don't choose to give that power. We move together organically, sometimes with close coordination, most often in a sort of friendly dance, our faces known to one another.

Several years ago a carpenter fell off a ladder, ending up paralyzed. A year after that an old community member who'd left years before moved home to die. More recently a tree fell on a car, killing a young child instantly. In all these cases, and many more, the community responded as a whole, yet with respect—giving time, money, benefit performances, auctions, and hot dishes. In a minor way, I've had ups and downs here, romances and breakups, that the community watched from an appropriate distance, neither judging nor meddling, reabsorbing me when the pain had passed. You could say this is what a good church does, but if you aren't part of the church you aren't always part of the circle of care. Here the island is a bit of a church itself. It has a spirit. It has a soul. If you "be" here "long," it takes you as one of its own.

Good Cheer

We have several community organizations that express that spirit. One is Good Cheer Food Bank. South Whidbey's first community charity started as a little food pantry in 1962. Approximately 20 percent of the families on the island use their services now, since the recession, but Good Cheer's mission isn't just a hunger-free community. It is to involve the community as volunteers, donors, and recipients. In other words, we are all part of a system that gives and gets and gives and gets until it's neither giving nor getting but community. Good Cheer raises money the normal way—fund-raising, begging, cajoling, etc.—but also through running three thrift stores "staffed" by 16 paid and 470 volunteer employees. Want to give back to the community? Volunteer at Good Cheer. Want to feel useful? Do the same. Want to end hunger, meet people, get out of the house, preview the merchandise as it comes through the door as donations? Good Cheer will "gainfully" employ you in serving.

The Good Cheer Food Bank used to be in the back room of their downtown Langley thrift store. Those in need, though, had to run the gauntlet of shoppers to get their week's food—an unnecessary embarrassment. Good Cheer raised a ton of money, bought the old Masonic Temple on a hill at a major crossroads, and converted it into a food distribution and merchandise-processing center. No more standard bags or boxes of standard food presented without choice. It looks like a grocery store, except that people pay with points rather than dollars. They have worked out a unique points system so that fresh produce and dairy are cheap and junk food is dear—just the opposite of the industrial system. Every person who needs food gets seventy points a month, with ten more points per additional family member. A ten-pound bag of potatoes is three points. So is a small box of instant mashed potatoes. A can of baked beans is three points, same as a two-pound bag of beans. Angel food cake mix is five points and limited to one per visit. A big bunch of kale or head of broccoli is one point. The points themselves make a point—healthy eating. Of course, if you buy dry beans or whole potatoes, you have to know how to cook. Good Cheer has cooking classes to teach people how to use the healthy ingredients. The crowning glory, though, is the .4-acre organic garden. Cary Peterson, a masterful gardener and Buddhist practitioner, organized hundreds of volunteers to build the garden. Dozens tend it, harvesting five thousand pounds of food a year. To provide fresh food for the table all year, Good Cheer now contracts with a young farming couple for winter vegetables.

Good Cheer has other sources of fresh food as well. The Gleeful Gleaners, who formed several years ago at a Transition Whidbey potluck, now add to the mountains of summer fruit, as does the Langley Middle School garden, The Whidbey Institute (a retreat center) garden, and the Greenbank Farm Training Center (more on that in the next chapter on my 50/50 diet). Farmers, gardeners, farmers' market vendors, egg ranchers, cattlemen, and fishermen often donate their surplus to the food bank as well.

This isn't instead of government programs. The food bank takes advantage of Northwest Harvest and Food Lifeline to purchase industrial food. They buy from Costco, get donations during food drives, and have couponing down to a science. But wherever the food comes from, the basic care that attaches to it is the same. Good Cheer is the essence of eating as belonging. Because you belong here, you will always have food.

Then a few years ago several women noticed an unseen group whose need for food wasn't being met—homeless teens. More than fifty, sometimes closer to a hundred, teens have run away from or gotten kicked out of their parents' homes and don't get enough to eat. So those caring women started W.I.N., Whidbey Island Nourishes. At first they simply put in refrigerators around the south end of the island so that teens, without having to beg or explain themselves, could pick up some healthy, fresh food every day. Eventually—thanks to a grant—they switched to vending machines reprogrammed to dispense without charge, yet with features that protect against food tampering. In addition, W.I.N. also sends lunches and snacks home every Friday with kids who normally rely on the school program. The people who pack these lunches love—I mean really love—W.I.N.

In a community of eaters, feeding one another is contagious. One person does it, others want to. Also, in a community of belonging, there is no sense of some being givers and others being getters. We are all part of here, giving and receiving.

While we here on South Whidbey tend to overcongratulate ourselves for how very cool we are, I am sure many readers live in communities like ours, communities where they have a sense of belonging, and so does anyone else who chooses to participate.

In the years ahead I'm certain that such communities will multiply. People will turn to one another as the cracks in the industrial system widen and more fall through. We will discover we are not falling into oblivion but rather into one another's arms. These stories are simply bread crumbs as you follow your own path to belonging somewhere, blessing the hands that feed *you*.

Is food love?

Am I simply saying that food is love, that I ingested love along with the turnips and greens? Yes, but even my understanding of "food is love" shifted. If I, as an anywhere eater, heard someone talk about food as love, I might have thought about a stereotypical Italian mama spooning seconds into her cringing bambino's bowl, sort of stuffing her family with food-love, like it or not. More likely, though, I would think of an eating disorder, food being used as a psychological substitute for a real-deal relationship. This substitution of food for love makes sense only in a society where food is abundant and distraction is epidemic, where love is difficult but ice cream is easy.

Geneen Roth is a cultural guru for those recovering from that food/love confusion. She nails it when she says on *Huffington Post,*

> During the first few bites, and before we get dazed by overeating, everything we want is possible. Everything we've lost is here now. And so we settle for the concrete version of our lost selves in the

form of food. And once food has become synonymous with goodness or love or fulfillment, you cannot help but choose it, no matter
how high the stakes are.

In her book *Women Food and God* she says,

> No matter what we weigh, those of us who are compulsive eaters
> have anorexia of the soul. We refuse to take in what sustains us. We
> live lives of deprivation. And when we can't stand it any longer, we
> binge. The way we are able to accomplish all of this is by the simple
> act of bolting—of leaving ourselves—hundreds of times a day.

"Anorexia of the soul." Trying to fill the need for love through putting
something in our body, or stripping some fat out! We starve ourselves when we are starved for love. Or we stuff ourselves when we
are starved for love.

I was clearly in some confusion about food and love when I started
the 10-mile diet. I'd just achieved Herculean weight loss so that I
might like my body again—and yet there I was ogling that table of
potluck dishes as though it were food porn. My 10-mile month didn't
change this. It simply gave me somewhere else to stand in relationship with food.

Now I am an eater in context, which is more satisfying by a long
shot than being two pants sizes smaller (though I do like that too!).

I love knowing that I am part of a food system that is all around
me, and actually doesn't stop at my skin. My belly is full of bacteria
chowing down on what I eat, helping me digest.

Nature doesn't really stop at some arbitrary property line—be it
my yard or my body. As I discovered, food isn't just what's in the
store or my garden. Edibles are everywhere. If I were quiet enough,
sensitive enough, I'd probably hear them. I am food to them as well.
Critters large and small would clean me up once I laid my body
down. Everything is food for something else. As my Amazon forest
experience long ago showed me: everything in the community of life

gives back to life—except the human. We are the species that hoards.

Clearly 99 percent of us don't live this way in North America. We treat most of the world as things to possess—cars, mates, jobs, degrees, houses replete with whirring machines to keep nature from intruding, rotting our food and our floors, melting our drywall. If humans suddenly departed, everything we do to hold nature at bay would be gone, allowing disintegration of the man-made world to process naturally. Everything is compost. We too, when we pass on.

Relational eating can bring us back to our senses—and back to a sense of gratitude. Our bodies are gifts; the "stuff" of us is just on loan from the Universe, due with interest (as in making something of ourselves) after four score and twenty years or so.

This is a bit much to contemplate with every bite, but relational eating reminds us that by eating we are participating in this web of relatedness by which we all live. It steps us back on a path to humility and to this alternately frightening and comforting thought that we are just a thread in the web of life, not the weaver.

Relational eating, then, serves as a touchstone for integrity. We vote with our eating. By purchasing the output of the industrial food system we are "buying it"—its processes and its assumptions. By eating local food, we tend our communities and nature. Being able to drive through a fast-food joint in our little personal tanks, protecting us from intrusion, gives us the sense of being a lone eater, but eating is never only a personal act.

Is even obesity, at least in part, an expression of the impersonality of our industrial food system? It disconnects food from real relationships with the hands and lands that feed us, allowing us to mindlessly consume it. If you are a relational eater, if you give love to your farmers by buying their food and receive love from your farmers by eating their food, gratitude itself could slow your hand-to-mouth repetitive-stress disorder.

As a relational eater, "food is love" signifies the love invested by every hand that feeds us—even the soil organisms that don't have hands per se. Such love arises from the natural relationship among the members of a living system. We all give that others may live. Our economic system drives us toward a zero-sum game, all competing to get more. A bit of reflection, though, reveals that if one actor in a system always wins, eventually there are no more losers for the winner to surpass. Game over, system collapse.

My friend Gary Vallat wrote me an e-mail about how his love for Duke and Kate LeBaron is knitted together with his weekly journey to buy their eggs.

I met Gary, an island newbie, when he moved here to be closer to his daughter and her family. He's a slender man, short silver hair, dark rimmed glasses, a Parkinson's tremor keeping his hands aflutter. We worked together on a project for Transition Whidbey and became friends, slowly discovering that we were both old idealists from the "back to the land" days.

Duke and Kate arrived in the mid-1980s at the tail end of the first wave of "back to the land" folks on the island. They built their own place, raised vegetables, animals, kids, and a bunch of hell in local politics. Duke was a big sober man, full of wisdom and knowledge won in that school of hard knocks called community organizing. Cancer had him by the ankle for nearly a decade and finally took him down in 2011, but not until he and Gary became friends, sharing conversations when Gary came to buy his weekly allotment of Duke and Kate's eggs, and fooling around with calculating the carrying capacity for the island (some people fool around this way).

After Duke's death, Gary wrote about those trips:

> The path to Duke's and Kate's property climbs a steep hill, follows a winding dirt road, crosses the fields of a remote residence (I had to connect with the neighbor to explain why I was "trespassing"). At Duke's back gate I am met by the donkey and the Navaho sheep who are always wary, sure that this interloper might endanger the regular meals they are accustomed to. They briefly announce their concern then flee with now visible uncertainty. I cross

the pasture and move through another gate passing the rooster's harem, berries and the raised bed farm. Beyond the next gate is the true guardian of the path, the goose . . . usually blowing the horn of attack, spreading wide the wings of retribution and going for my ankles. Closing the final gate I arrive at the massive door to the castle where the prince waits in his chambers.

Now the prince is gone but the path is still there, leading to memories and his partner who is willing from time to time to join me in bringing Duke back to life. . . . Kate brings out her cookies, puts the kettle on the gas stove and puts another log on the fire in the wood cook stove so that we can share our stories and complete a connection built on the memory of food—and Duke.

"The memory of food—and Duke." This is the wholeness of relational eating. The visit to Duke's widow, the "grocery shopping," the wander across a hill (violating conventions of private property), and successfully negotiating the gauntlet of animals, all of this is "eggs." It is kindness, hunger, nutrition, being outdoors, being threaded into the web of life (some of it braying), the warm fire, the tea, the triumphant walk home with one's booty in a backpack. And from this relationship with Duke arose a comfort in sitting with the ill and dying that led to a new engagement with the local hospice. It is stepping into the river of community, surrendering, allowing oneself to be part of a wholeness while still being Gary or Vicki or Duke or Kate or the goose spreading her wings. How wonderful to live somewhere that receives one's love. How wonderful to know that eating is belonging.

Eating Together

What would relational eating be without relationships? Even though I live alone I find ways to dine with others—sometimes simply bringing my own plate of food over to a friend's house so we can enjoy a family meal. But the natural response to relational eating is gratitude. This can be as simple as saying grace over every meal, no matter how many specific links in the supply chain you can name.

I learned the following grace when I was part of a team that met monthly to develop a training that would help people change. Each weekend we'd take a break from the intensity of our brainstorming to eat. We'd hold hands and say the Buddhist blessing:

> *This food is the gift of the whole universe—the earth, the sky, and much hard work.*
> *May we live in a way that makes us worthy to receive it.*
> *May we transform our unskillful states of mind, especially our greed.*
> *May we take only foods that nourish us and prevent illness.*
> *We accept this food so that we may realize the path of practice.*[1]

Grace before a meal and bedtime prayers were common when I was little. I don't know what's happened to "Now I lay me down to sleep, I pray the Lord my soul to keep . . ." but I can venture a guess about mealtime prayers. How many singles with no hands to hold still say grace when they sit down to eat? How has this changed our sense of eating, from being a relational act to being a distracted act, reading a book or clicking through e-mails as we chew and swallow?

Only the most devout among us follow the prayer cycles of traditional religions. Orthodox Jews are traditionally required to say a hundred blessings a day. Explanations vary as to why, but so what? Blessing opportunities abound. Put in a modern context, traditional cycles of daily prayer can translate into spontaneous *berakhot* (blessings) for every and any amazing moment when you recognize God hiding out in daily life. You can say a blessing when your eyes fly open in the morning, and when you wash your hands and face. You can appreciate as you dress that every limb articulates (more or less). In the same way you can say supermarket blessings for jars of peanut butter and for bins of chocolate-covered almonds and for whoever butchered that chicken, skinned it, boned it, placed it in a Styrofoam tray with something akin to a menstrual pad for any ooze, pulled taut the plastic, and slapped on a label with a bar code. If that weren't enough amazement, what about the good intentions of the chemists who figured out those preservatives we now revile. Dollars to doughnuts—as they say—these men and women really thought they were bringing us better living through chemistry.

In fact I do take such prayers with me when shopping, gardening, cooking, and eating. I shop in the Star Store with such gratitude. The cans and bins and wrapped meats and deli and paper products are *a gift of the whole universe, the earth, the sky, and much hard work*. In between conversations with friends by the cheese and between the fruits and nuts, I remind myself what a miracle it is that all this food is mine for a brief swipe of a debit card.

Back in the day when interviewers asked me for my top money-saving tip, I'd often say: "Gratitude." It's very hard to impulse-buy when you are awash in gratitude for everything you have, which includes not just this shirt but *the earth, the sky, and the much hard work* of the generations who brought you the comforts of this life, just as it is.

It seems to be that way for relational eating. Even all this time later, hard to zone out with a spoon without thinking about the hands that are feeding me, without recognizing the preciousness of food.

Relational Farming

It stands to reason, once you think about it, that you can't be a relational eater without relational farmers—farmers in relationship with seeds, land, seasons, and more.

The closer your farmers are to the soil, the more they are your link to blessing the earth that feeds you.

The "farmer" has many faces: hunter/gatherer, subsistence farmers who own land, tenant farmers who rent land, truck farmers who bring crops to market as they mature, subscription farmers who grow for specific customers (CSAs or restaurants), family farmers who still grow a diversity of crops and livestock, industrial farmers who are more like industrialists than farmers—who hire farmworkers to actually do the work.

Whom you choose as the farmer for each product you buy—in the supermarket or farmers' market—gives you a different relationship with the soil. Knowing your farmer means you are only one step removed from this humus (healthy soil), a word that shares a root with *human* and *humane* and *humble*.

By contrast, buying industrial food puts you in relationship with a faraway soil-like substance, diminished of life but bulked up with soil "steroids." The foodlike substances are half laboratory creations, with added flavors and stabilizers and genes for cold or poison tolerance.

Stepping into Your Farmer's Boots

The closer you are to your farmer, the more you see through her eyes and share his challenges.

You become sensitized to what he or she deals with daily in producing local food in an industrial system.

You see how the USDA and FDA, while protecting consumers from bad apples (so to speak) among industrial producers, regulate the life right out of small-scale producers who want to sell their surplus to their neighbors. Some trade is simply against the law. I bought Elsie's milk from Belinda and got goat cheese from Nina like I used to score marijuana. Both acts were illegal and therefore could not be spoken about. When we'd see each other around town, we couldn't speak out loud about . . . ahem . . . that.

Some of my farmers have worked around these restrictions by forming co-ops—owning a piece of a cow or a goat and therefore milking "their" animal legally.

Some products are constrained by legislation requiring permits, inspections, licenses—all adding cost to the product—too much cost for small-scale operations.

Vicky Brown of Little Brown Farm is a case in point. Another islander, Lynn Swanson, finally got her sheep dairy licensed, but at this writing Vicky runs the only remaining legal dairy on the island, milking her herd of twenty-two goats every day. The playing field between her cheese and anywhere cheese—goat, sheep, or cow—is so unlevel she'd have few customers if she hadn't cultivated local loyalists at the farmers' market and upscale wine shops. She turns the milk from her "ladies" into yummy handcrafted cheeses that she has to sell for top dollar—six times what bottom-dollar cheese fetches—because of the many dollars she has to spend to comply with all the regulations and inspections and pay all the licensing and insurance to sell her wares legally. I've stood in her barn, each of us nuzzling a baby doe with ears softer than my cat's back. I've looked around as she pointed out the special stalls and paints and bathrooms and sinks she has had to install to comply with regulations. She's run the numbers for me, punctuating the recitation with a snort at the people who ask why her cheese is so expensive.

Could she simply skip the rules and sell raw milk cheese in the underground food trading system that flourishes here via friendship networks? Of course, but then she would not be Vicky Brown who takes pride in her one and only profession—dairywoman. She left a high-paid corporate job—bringing with her all her professional skills—to build a real business and succeed. She is, therefore, on the front lines of confronting the unfairness of a system that does not make any allowance for scale of operations. A license is a license, no matter what size your herd. Inspection fees are inspection fees, no matter what size your operation.

The same playing-field tilt discourages people from buying five-dollars-a-pound chicken and Georgina's grain and Georgie's beans (at least five times the price of their industrial counterparts). This is not just a question of scale. Migrant labor and undocumented laborers earn a pittance and have little voice in shifting their conditions. Factory food isn't necessarily cheaper to produce than artisan food because some of the costs are hidden in our taxes. In addition to the low price we pay for it directly at the market, we also pay indirectly through Big Farm subsidies, environmental cleanup from shoddy practices, or the health costs of food-borne illnesses. With local food, we pay premium price because our farmer does not have those subsidies and does not take cheaper shortcuts that could endanger the environment and our health.

Many locals get around complying with costly regulations by trading in a person-to-person food system. Hundreds of people on this island raise animals for home consumption. They can sell a quarter or half of an animal to me legally, but not cuts of meat. To get a USDA certification on an island that has no abattoir means animals are either slaughtered in a very expensive USDA-approved mobile slaughter unit or loaded onto a truck to go to the closest USDA-approved slaughterhouse on the mainland. Several farmers, including the Long family and 3 Sisters on the north end of the island, do go this route, complying with USDA regulations as part of the "Whidbey Island Grown" brand that is slowly entering the marketplace. But a lot of hyperlocal meat here is traded in the relational web. In August, as I looked for 10-mile meat and milk, I actually dived beneath the surface of the food system into this web of relationships. I now know that hundreds of other people are like me: they know who grows their meat, milk, eggs, and veggies. By name. And know their kids' names. And show up to help when times are hard.

Can My Exotics Be Relational?

What about food from afar? Is that relational food? In the sense that we are all part of the web of life on this planet, every mouthful is a relational act. We are ingesting the hard work of every hand that touched the food from field to store, the migrant workers, the truckers, the two A.M. shelf stockers, the checker. It is harder to feel these relationships, though. They aren't our literal neighbors; they don't sit in church with us, or attend our performances, or send their kids to our schools. Accountability is more abstract with anywhere eating, but with local or regional eating your integrity is visible to everyone.

In fact, relational eating can lead us to a food ethic that governs every mouthful. Our food choices support healthy soils, family farms, thriving communities, fair labor practices, good agricultural practices, fresh air, and conservation—or not. Local is where you are accountable. All food is local somewhere. What's life like for my lemon grower? Do the pickers in the olive groves for my olive oil have enough to eat? Where does my coffee come from and what natural systems were mowed down for those beans to grow?

Relational eating, then, is exiting the revolving doors of the anonymous food courts of the world and entering a web of nourishing relationships where your eating is both receiving (great food!)—and giving (caring for the life and lot of your farmers). It is personal—eating for flavor, freshness, purity, health. And it is political—understanding that where you spend your food dollars is a vote for the health of the earth.

What If I Just Want to Buy the Food, Not Befriend the Farmer?

You can buy local food without being a relational eater—and still do a bushel of good. You can—and many do—keep an industrial food mind-set while buying local food. You can treat your CSA like a grocery delivery service rather than a chance to invest in a farmer, sharing the risks and rewards of the season. You can treat the farmers' market like a produce department, not realizing as you squeeze the fruit that the farmer in front of you nurtured that tomato from seed, picked it at peak ripeness, and offers it to you with love. You can comparison shop too, cruising the stalls for the best buys. It's an understandable way to behave in an industrial food world, but odd in a relational world. You can pick up your eggs or flowers from the farm stand, drop in your money, and never see the hands that picked them for you. These transactions are not transformational—but they are still likely good for you, good for the local economy, and good for the environment.

So yes, you can buy local food without any intention of making new friends or being such a stick in the mud that you start to grow roots, branches, and leaves.

Why Buy Local?

The following is my list of very good reasons—in addition to relational eating—for buying local food. I've tested them all in my own experience, but they are not "the gospel truth." Chew on them for yourself, swallowing only what makes real sense to you.

This list can be a starting point for making local food part of your diet of beliefs and practices as well as what you eat. Is local food really fresher, tastier, more nourishing, more just, more expensive but worth it, and beneficial for local economies? The important thing is to develop your own relationship with food and the hands that feed you—and my observations might be a motivation to do that.

Seven Very Good Personal Reasons to Eat Local Food

Fresh!

The fresher the food, the more nutritious and delicious it is. No one who has eaten a sun-warmed tomato would argue with that. But let's take a deeper look. While "local" is a distance measure, "fresh" is a time measure. If you—or your farmer—harvest food in the morning and eat it by bedtime, it's really fresh! If you don't eat the fresh-picked food right away, though, it doesn't compete with anywhere produce, picked and packed at peak halfway around the world and, through an amazing feat of logistics, stocked in your grocery store by dinnertime the next day. Nor does it compete with flash-frozen-in-the-fields fruits and veggies. So local increases the likelihood of fresh —but you have to eat fresh, not just buy fresh.

Ripe!

Much of the produce in your market looks fresh-picked, but it might have been picked green and ripened later with ethylene gas. Peak ripeness is when the nutrients are in the highest concentration. Think about it from the fruit's point of view. It's that final burst of energy to make the best seed possible before the season ends. It's the pinnacle, you might say, of the plant's creative energies, giving its all before dying. Because local fruits are more likely vine- or tree-ripened, they may be imbued with that extra burst of energy, extra sweetness, juiciness, and nutritional richness. As such, they may be a day away from rotting, which is why square, flavorless tomatoes gained favor—no taste but boy do they last!

Tasty!

Yes, delicious can be a very good reason to go local. Besides taste from freshness, local gardeners and farmers are able to grow more flavorful varieties that don't stand up to the rigors of monocropping and shipping, that go from ripe to perfect to rotten in a few short days, that are super sweet or thin-skinned or oddly shaped. They can grow varieties bred over time, not in laboratories, to the precise combination of sun, rainfall, and soils of your valley, not the valley a few hundred miles south. As you eat a wider variety of apples or potatoes or greens, you really do start to distinguish between the flavors and textures. Eating the limited varieties of each fruit or vegetable grown by an industrial food system has dulled our "sniffer." We no longer need taste to determine if something is good for us—the USDA assures us that we can eat whatever is sold in the store. Yes, 99 percent of the time they are right but we've outsourced a natural instinct to computer tracing systems. Encountering novel fresh foods grown around you may awaken your taste buds—and the flavors may be richer as well.

Wholesome!

Unless you live near a junk-food factory, local food (whether 10- or 100-mile) would tend to come to you in its unadulterated, unprocessed form. To paraphrase Popeye, "A yam is a yam." And squash is squash and tomatoes are tomatoes and wheat is ground fresh and baked into a hearty loaf. You are less likely to consume toxins, additives, food coloring, stabilizers, and a host of other extras that you get in highly processed foods.

My friend Suzanne decided to make whole, unprocessed, and unpackaged foods the focus of her Lenten practice. It didn't have to be local so she had a wide variety of whole foods to pick from, but getting even whole foods home without putting them in plastic was a challenge. Like me, she discovered that fidelity to that values-imposed food constraint required a lot of attention in the beginning and then, by Easter, had simply become the way she ate. Along the way she saw, as I had, how complex and adulterated our food system has become. She brought used containers for food from the bulk bins, bought plenty of produce, and got her chicken right from the butcher's big delivery box before it was plastic-wrapped in the store. She got behind the *Wizard of Oz* screen and entered relational eating—at the very least with the butcher and bulk food buyers at the grocery store.

Frugal!

You heard that right. After all of my belly-aching about the cost of a chicken, how can I say local food saves you money? Cary Peterson of the Good Cheer Garden teaches classes on effective, productive backyard gardening, called Growing Groceries, so that the people who use the food bank (and anyone else) can supplement their income with this other kind of green stuff. In one Internet article I saw, the author claimed seven hundred dollars' worth of food on a ten-by-ten-foot plot. Such stories are all over the Web. Gardeners love to tell how they did it. When the going gets expensive, the frugal get growing.

Rebellion!

Occupy your food system! If you want to protest the creep of corporate control over what we hold dear—our food supply, democracy, justice, dignity—then eat local food. Withdraw your agreement with the industrial food system by withdrawing your participation to whatever degree you can consistent with your health and sanity. Integrity comes when your actions are aligned with your intentions and your values. Sometimes you just eat what's available as you work for whatever cause "works" your soul, but local food can be a powerful tool for walking your talk. Or I should say, eating your talk. As I discovered in February, you could substitute local foods for 50 percent of your anywhere foods and still eat like a queen. Some go to extremes on this—growing all their own food and shunning anything from the industrial system. The rest of us will stir up small rebellions in our purchasing and cooking and dining.

Freedom!

Rebellion—protesting a system you abhor—is political. But freedom—liberating yourself from the shackles of whatever you let control you—is spiritual. Seed, soil, sunlight, and water offer you freedom from dependency and freedom to participate in feeding yourself. If you cannot grow your own food, if you don't know any farmers whose food you can buy, if you are utterly dependent on supermarkets and takeout, then you are a prisoner of the industrial food system. Eating local food puts your money into nourishing local production for local consumption. It frees you and your community from unnecessary dependencies.

Seven Reasons Why We as a Society Should Eat Local Food

Fertility

Once embarked on my local food quest, I wanted to expand my own gardening knowledge. I attended a class on biodynamic farming, expecting a lecture on techniques but getting an hour lecture on "fertility," which is, the lecturer said, a byproduct of the natural vitality of the life of the soil. We don't *put* fertility *into* soil; soil has it and we just have to encourage it. We cooperate with fertility by making a hospitable home for soil critters and water flow and sun, by treating the soil well. Most industrial farming diminishes fertility . . . and then uses fossil fuel to manufacture "fertilizer." But the earth is naturally fertile. As life cycles through it, the fertility even increases! I realized I no longer thought about land as fertile. I thought about fertilizing land, either through chemicals or compost. I thought of fertility as an additive, not as a characteristic of life. I presumed fertility gets used up, and needs to be topped off by human intervention. But this biodynamic teacher turned everything on its head. Fertility is not scarce; it is everywhere.

Biodynamic farmers work with the fertility of the land through love and attention—as well as cow manure and special kinds of biodynamic preparations. Small-scale farmers who serve their communities, family farmers who grow for their regions, build the fertility of their soils through tending, through relationship. It may not be certified organic soil—as I said earlier, the little guy often deems certification too costly and their loyal customers know their practices are organic—but it is "relational soil," teeming with life. These soil organisms are the ultimate "farm animals." When you buy local food you are supporting farmers who support the fertility of their land. If people in community everywhere did the same, we would, from the bottom up, green the earth.

Security

Your local food supply cannot easily be disrupted by terrorism. It wouldn't even be on the enemy's radar—it's too small a target. It wouldn't likely be curtailed by supply-chain failures or tainted by botulism (well, if you don't take care with canning you can do this to yourself, but you'd know before you opened the jar). Unless your microclimate takes an irremediable turn for the worse, your food supply won't be choked off due to climate events. Recall the story of food riots in Mozambique when Russia stopped exporting wheat after an unprecedented heat wave ignited fires, burning much of their crop.

Rising oil prices might also impact your food security. The debate is not whether we'll run through the easy and cheap oil and be left with the difficult to exploit and costly oil—it's just when this will happen and what will replace it.

We the eaters of the United States have little comprehension of what peak oil means for our daily bread. Oil is everywhere in the industrial food system. It runs our farm machinery—tractors, seeders, weeders, harvesters, combines, and even airplanes to spray the herbicides and pesticides. It is the raw material for fertilizer and many other agricultural chemicals. It is used as a fuel for picking, processing, packaging, shipping, and delivery to stores we get to in our cars. What a miracle. What a victory for human cleverness. Yet what a vulnerability.

When Russia cut oil exports in half after the 1990 collapse of the

Soviet Union, Cuba's economy went into a tailspin. Their fossil-fuel-intensive food system nearly collapsed, and the nation mobilized to grow food in every square inch of the cities.

The good news from Cuba is that necessity was the mother of a great deal of creativity and community. With the strength of government mandates and their own ingenuity, Cubans transitioned from a highly mechanized, industrial agricultural system to one using organic methods of farming and local, urban gardens. They didn't go all the way back to the horse and plow—they used fuel precisely where it was needed and applied their ingenuity to finding elegant ways to produce ample food using traditional methods. They moderated their expectations too—becoming less enslaved to the "more is better" mind-set. And they worked. And they ate less. And they lost weight. And they were still plenty healthy, aided by establishing—in their times of constraint, even—universal health care. They became a people working together, and they survived.

Relational eating, being an "eater-in-community," can settle our fears about being fed on every level. When you have no relationship with food other than the megamart, you seem well supplied but are helpless without that store. When you stand in the middle of a living food system, growing some, trading some, buying some local and some from afar, you have more power to assure that you are fed—and fed well. Relational eating doesn't necessarily mean local food; it means that you, the eater, understand your place in the world.

Local Prosperity

Buy Local campaigns ask people to spend their national currency locally, circulating dollars through their neighbors' wallets rather than through the coffers of distant multinational corporations. Local farmers are businesses, so spending your dollars with them means those same dollars will probably pass through the tills of the feed store, the local restaurants, the local thrift store, and more. Some say money is like manure—it's good only if you spread it around. Buying from local growers fertilizes the local economy. This is good.

Farmland

Preserving agricultural lands—keeping them from becoming shopping plazas or strip malls—requires more than individual eaters putting their mouths on the line. Your eating a local rutabaga doesn't of itself do anything to protect farmland, but it is likely to increase your commitment to preserving farmland (through investing, donating, volunteering, advocating, activism, organizing) now that you recognize how crucial it is to your well-being. In the industrial mind-set, farmland is like everything else: invisible and someone else's responsibility. We imagine rolling fields and red barns, and small blond children in pinafores running in the meadow with dandelions held high like pinwheels. The closest we get to this bucolic image, though, is a Sunday drive in the country—or playing the Internet game FarmVille.

In communities across North America, organizations are working to keep farmland out of development and in agricultural productivity. For example, the Ebey's Landing National Historical Reserve on Whidbey Island resulted from a unique partnership to preserve prime farmland, working farms, and the history of farming on the island. Likewise, the Marin Agricultural Land Trust in California raises money to conserve farmland, protecting it from development. I found that making a commitment to local food soon leads to the "hard stuff"—finding mechanisms to protect farmland and support farmers. At this writing I have one loan out to a farmer; payback is scheduled for three years and I'm taking my interest in vegetables. My community has developed an innovative lending mechanism— relocalizing is becoming everyone's business.

Bringing this issue really close to home, I live on the edge of a few of the original local farms. The town has crept up the hill from the water's edge, yet several pastures remain where sheep, horses, and cows graze and hay is cut in the summer. When the matriarch of one of the families finally passed away in 2005, and it was possible that their farm would also pass, into a subdivision, the family instead chose to make it a community asset. Dorothy Anderson, granddaughter of Anders and Bertine Anderson, who arrived in Langley in 1907, set aside a chunk of her family's twenty acres to be used for the city's first community garden. Dorothy is having the time of her life bringing life back to the farm. (There are now goats, steer, and a large field cultivated by Chris Korrow, a biodynamic farmer.) If she had her druthers, we'd all move up there and live together. Talk about relational farming! But mechanisms exist to help owners of farmland to harvest money from their property without selling to developers.

Waste

Both the emotional investment in relational eating and the money investment in buying local makes you far less inclined to waste food.

The industrial system has no such signals. In fact, the more food you buy (whether you eat it or not), the more profit for the producers. If food is cheap, waste is easy.

American per capita food waste increased to more than fourteen hundred calories per person per day in 2009, an increase of approximately 50 percent since 1974. According to Jonathan Bloom, author of *American Wasteland:*

> We don't eat 25% of the food we buy. We throw away $2,200 each year in uneaten food, from spoilage and plate waste
> 97% of discarded food ends up in landfills, producing methane, a greenhouse gas 25 times more heat trapping than CO_2
> 20% of edible meat ends up in landfills.[2]

From the *Ecocentric* blog I learned more useful—albeit overly simplified—ways to frame the issue, including:

- Because we use 10 units of fossil energy to produce one unit of food energy, feeding the population requires 10 percent of the total annual U.S. energy consumption.[3]
- If we wasted just 5 percent less food, it would be enough to feed 4 million Americans; 20 percent less waste could feed 25 million Americans annually.[4]

According to Marian Nestle, author, nutritionist, and professor at New York University:

> Our version of capitalism requires companies to grow and report growth to Wall Street every 90 days. This puts the pressure on short-term, not longer-term, profits. I see that as at the root of a great deal of difficulty in the obesity problem. If companies have to grow, they're going to have to produce and sell more food, not less. But all of them can't succeed in that because we already have too much food—3,900 calories per day per capita in the US, twice the average need. . . . They can make better food, but it doesn't sell as well, it's more expensive to make, and those cheap food products are immensely profitable.[5]

This is not just a North American problem; an equal amount of food is also wasted in less-developed countries because it rots in the fields or on the way to market.

Local food does nothing about that problem, but it promotes food conservation.

Kids

Healthy school lunches are now beyond a good idea; they are a shared cause. Alice Waters, who pioneered the use of fresh local ingredients at Chez Panisse in Berkeley, is now pushing for edible school yards where kids get their hands in the dirt, learn about the cycles of life, and put fresh very local food on their lunchroom tables. There are stories like hers all over the country. On Whidbey, teacher Kimmer Morris organized the garden at Langley Middle School so students could learn to garden and love produce; they also send hundreds of pounds of fresh produce to the food bank. Ann Cooper calls herself the renegade lunch lady. She started her quest to combat childhood obesity by serving Long Island kids regional, organic, seasonal, sustainable food—and is now a passionate speaker, writer, author, and crusader for healthy school lunches, struggling against the mighty forces of pink slime (a heat and ammonia-gas-processed beef slaughter byproduct added to some ground beef) and chicken nuggets and ketchup as a vegetable. If you experience the food from your local farmers as more wholesome, nutritious, and delicious than industrial food, you'll want to support kids eating it as well.

The Future!

If you have a concern about the effects of the triple crisis on the generations who will inhabit the earth once we are gone, you want with all your heart to leave this world better than you found it. I've lived that value through my activism, figuratively doing chin-ups on the overconsumption bar trying to lower our collective impact. This has been rewarding and exhausting. I've also run personal experiments in sustainability—and written about it—as well as worked on changing the mind-set of the culture from "more" to "enough." Maybe you, like me, have battled the forces of decline and are tuckered out, though still in the game. My shift to local food has both settled me down and fired me up. Because I am now grounded and I have energy to give. My work is not abstract—a response to information. My energy doesn't just come from fear or anger—it comes from the actual food as well as the relationships that sustain me.

We've all talked a blue streak about the need for change—and God bless the talkers because they awaken the people. But for me the relational farmers are primary builders of wealth for the generations. Perhaps now, as I approach seventy, I am more aware of the fact that others will inherit the earth. I'm just a word farmer. As a gardener, I dabble. As a local eater, I'm partial but at least aware and intentional. Yet tending my life toward relational eating allows me to be carried along toward the end of my life with great satisfaction. Local food has been a doorway into greater security than I could ever have by buying long-term-care insurance. I am my community's long-term-care insurance, and I'm beginning to really trust that they will be there for me as needed.

You and I don't need to be farmers to get our Girl Scout badge in local food. There are so many ways eaters can influence the future of farming.

We can get politically active. In the next chapter I'll talk more about my own search for policies that support young farmers and policies that liberate local small-scale growers from some of the regulations designed to assure the wholesomeness of industrial food. Your issues may be different, but if you simply pick one farmer to care about, and eat their food while learning about their joys and challenges, you will be on a similar hunt for solutions.

We can put our money where our mouths are—literally. We can invest in local or regional farms. Jason Bradford, an early relocalization activist, has partnered with a venture capitalist to reclaim abused farmland in the Bay Area and systematically return it to health. They are laser-focused, numbers-oriented, unsentimental, on a mission, and intending to profit, but they are also committed to implementing the best science-based organic farming practices they know. We can facilitate farm loans for small producers who want to innovate; the Local Investing Opportunity Network (LION) model currently spreading in the Pacific Northwest is one mechanism. It's not an investing club. It's an investing network that connects people who want to invest locally with local businesspeople—including farmers—with projects that need $1,000—or $100,000. The network merely facilitates meeting. Beyond that the lenders and borrowers are on their own to make whatever deals they want. We just started one here on Whidbey, called W.I.L.L. (Whidbey Island Local Lending). You hear it coming . . . "Where there is a W.I.L.L. there is a way." Or you can donate money through organizations like Kickstarter. Vicky Brown, our local goat milkmaid, ran a successful Kickstarter campaign to expand her business. Or you can help farmers research what government grants might be available to them.

If we are businesspeople ourselves, we can notice opportunities and build businesses that support local growers, like food hubs. According to the USDA a food hub is "a centrally located facility with a business management structure facilitating the aggregation, storage,

processing, distribution, and/or marketing of locally/regionally produced food products." Some are teaching centers as well. Some are
associated with commercial kitchens where people can turn their
dollar-a-pound produce into five-dollars-a-pound chutneys, sauces,
and soups. On Whidbey there are several new businesses as of this
writing. A lavender farmer is opening a dry-pack facility—open to
the public—where she can package her lavender rather than shipping
it out of state to a packer. A group is discussing buying a grain mill
and putting it into very visible operation so grain growers can grind
the emmer, kamut, wheat, and barley they've grown; local bakers can
work with fresh-ground flours; and local eaters can make nutritious
cracked-grain cereals. As small enterprises, they may flourish or die
on the vine, but they are indicators of this fertile climate for local business development.

Is any of this easy? Nope. We're dealing with human beings here,
and business partnerships of all sorts are fraught with challenges. Yet
investing in local agriculture is a financial way to support local food
beyond your willingness to pay a little extra for those beets, squash,
and chickens.

We can be educators as well—as I am doing now. We can form
and work for nonprofits that support local farming. We can frequent
restaurants that take pains to serve as much local food as possible.
Jess Dowdell, formerly of Ca'buni café, housed in the Mukilteo Coffee roasting warehouse, is starting a new catering venture. For sure
I'll stop there for sandwiches. Pickles Deli has a local menu. All the
chefs and farmers who contributed recipes are committed to using
local ingredients.

Is local food a miracle cure? No. It takes time. It challenges your
habits and abilities. Your local dollars spent at the farmers' market
could as well go into a purchase at a big box store as into your local
barber's pocket. It may not be more nutritious if it's many days old or
grown in depleted soil. As a commitment to address big global issues, it's truly a drop in the bucket. Unless you grow your own in
abundance, you are likely spending more money. As for relational

eating, what if you don't really like your farmers after all? What if you like the idea of local food but not the fact of it happening next door—with a quack quack here and a hee-haw there and a manure pile by your fence. Local food. But NIMBY (not in my backyard).

No, local is not the new black. Or green. It is, however, a lens that brings a lot into focus, and it is right at hand, actionable, and beneficial, at least to your farmers. It is a point of entry into making a difference in very earthy (I can't say concrete) ways.

For me the most profound result of a commitment to local is leaving a legacy of hope and health and, in my lifetime, enjoying the benefits of belonging to a place and a people—the security and love and mutual aid.

Relational eating—eating as an act of belonging—is what I offer you, along with these dozen other motivations that now seem true enough to me to base my life on them.

Now What?

Having wrestled with all these questions and issues, with my inner comfort-food demons, with how I cling to frugality, with my preferences for convenience, and with my desire to relegate food to basically inexpensive refueling for a busy life, I finally surrendered my right to food ignorance. Now when I eat, I understand the web of relationships that brought this food to my lips and the web of relationships I am developing by which hands I choose to feed me. I understand this viscerally, emotionally, and ethically.

While it may seem easier in the short run to just grab a burger and drive on, I think the freedom of being awake is in the long run more satisfying.

So I am inviting you to look under the hood of industrial eating to recognize what it is not giving you and invest some life energy in building up around you a food system that gives you what's missing.

Now It's Your Turn

What motivates you to change?

It's time to ask yourself whether and how you might want to shift your eating closer to home. I've shared my long list of benefits for eating locally. Of course for me the linchpin was relational eating—how eating the food grown by my community made me part of that community. Belonging, for me, is not just a warm fuzzy feeling; the place is ever more the grounding force in my life—where I come from when I venture into the world, where I return to to be restored.

From that core, all the many other benefits radiate for me. Your core might be different. Your motivations to start might be different. So here's a self-test to see what might move you to make the local shift. Rate each item on a scale of 1–10, with 1 being "not for me," 5 being "I'll try anything once," and 10 being "absolutely yes."

Possible Motivation for Local Eating

- *Curiosity*—I want to learn about myself, my food habits, and the food system. _____
- *Health*—I want to be healthier, and local brings me fresh, nutritious food. _____
- *Fresh*—I love fresh food and don't care for packaged and processed food. _____
- *Financial*—It's worth the extra money, and by growing and trading I can afford it. _____
- *Accessible*—I care that everyone has fresh food in their neighborhood. _____
- *Safety*—I trust my local growers more than I trust the industrial system that brings us such delights as E. coli and mad cow disease. I want food free of GMOs, toxins, antibiotics, herbicides, and pesticides. _____
- *Security*—I want to know that I and those I love will have enough to eat if/when food supply chains fracture or are financially not feasible. _____

- *Sovereignty*—I want to take back control of my food from the corporate system. _____
- *Soil*—I want to rebuild conditions for fertility in our soils and water. _____
- *Seed*—I want to participate in preservation of genetic heritage. _____
- *Nature*—I want to be in nature, protect nature, understand nature. _____
- *Competency*—I want to be self-reliant—to learn to cook, garden, raise animals, forage, and fish. The more skills I have, the safer I feel. _____
- *Climate change*—I want to think now about how climate change affects me and my community, and set up adaptive systems. _____
- *Peak oil*—I want to support alternatives to the current fossil-fuel-intensive form of agriculture. _____
- *Justice*—I want to help assure that everyone in my community has access to healthy, affordable, and abundant food. _____
- *Children*—I want our children to have healthy, nontoxic, plentiful food. _____
- *Care for the generations to come*—I want to assure that our grandchildren will have healthy, accessible, affordable, and abundant food. _____
- *Belonging*—I want to put down roots where I live and be part of a community. _____
- *Ethics*—I want the impact of my eating to be a blessing for others and the earth. _____
- *Community*—I want to strengthen the ties of community. _____

TOTAL _____

Where to Begin

If your total number is over 125, I'd say it's worth picking someplace to begin and giving it a try. You can begin with any of the following:

- What you grow: even sprouts.
- Where you shop: Try a farmers' market, farm stand, or CSA in addition to your regular stores.
- What you buy: Pick at least one food to buy from your region. Pick a local producer—perhaps a baker or a soup maker—and buy their product no matter where the ingredients come from.
- What you don't buy: Avoid overfished species, factory-raised animals, nonorganic produce.
- How you spend your money: Invest in local food to build your local food system.
- What you eat: Learn what grows well in your area and base some meals around those foods.
- How you cook: Cook from scratch with what's on hand. Learn to use a pressure cooker.
- Whom you eat with: Increase your sit-down meals with others.
- How your meat is grown: pasture-raised, organic feed.
- How much you eat: Moderate your eating in honor of the life embodied in your meal.
- What you order in restaurants: Look for words like *local, catch of the day, seasonal.*
- What you choose for a career: Does it help in any way to regenerate the vitality of regional food systems?
- What you advocate for in your school, workplace, place of worship: Influence your networks to eat simple, local foods; influence your food-service people to grow and serve more local foods.
- How you vote: Understand issues affecting small-scale regional farmers and farming and vote for candidates who advocate for these.
- What you say: Write or speak about local food; stick up for it.

Meaning to do everything, we often do nothing. Thinking the task is big, we often don't begin. Begin with just one step, though, something that appeals to you, and you enter into change. Who knows where that will lead?

My Shopping Criteria

I like to buy what is grown locally . . . by someone I know . . . who probably sends her kids to local schools . . . frequents local restaurants . . . and maybe acts in plays or plays in a jazz ensemble or calls square dances. I put my community at the center of my eating.

This means I also eat with the seasons as much as possible, and will do my own canning and freezing to have those same pleasures off-season.

I like to "reward" with my dollars regional producers who are pioneering local production of a food I like. I get my raw milk from a regional legal dairy. I buy regional grains and beans if possible and baked goods from regional bakeries that favor regional flours. I can't always stomach the price differential, but I know my values and inch toward integrity.

When the price is right I buy organic when I can't buy local—"right" for me being under twice as expensive. It's my investment in soil. Many friends choose organic no matter what the cost. I'll get there. Eventually.

I buy my staples—beans, grains, oils, spices, nuts—in bulk rather than prepackaged. Yes, I reuse my plastic bags and bottles when possible so I'm as close as I can get to simply taking handfuls of whole foods home.

I avoid, if possible, GMO commodities. I'm not convinced that fish genes in tomatoes will kill me, but I am convinced that the industrial commodity system is decimating soils, cultures, tastes, natural genetic lines, and small farmers.

I favor whole foods wherever they are grown.

I look for fair trade coffee and chocolate and exotics.

I use the sustainable harvest list for fish.[6]

I buy pasture-raised meat within my region if possible.

I refer to the Environmental Working Group list for the dirty dozen most toxic vegetables. This year it's apples, celery, strawberries, peaches, spinach, nectarines (imported), grapes (imported), sweet bell peppers, potatoes, blueberries, lettuce, kale, and collard greens.[7]

When there is no ethical difference between product A and product B, I let my frugality be my guide.

I forage when I can—and this sometimes includes a dignified conversation with a produce manager about where he's sending all those vegetable trimmings and rejects, after which I've been known to take home a bag.

And when all else fails—or when my willingness flags—I simply do what I want, knowing my wants have been educated by my good habits.

If I bump into you at a fast-food joint sometime, it doesn't mean I've fallen off the wagon. Since you are there too, sit down and join me.

Try These Recipes

Here are recipes from Jess and local fine chef Sieb Jurriaans of Primo Bistro. The Bistro's deck is the place to dine in the summer. You are on First Street, overlooking Saratoga Passage, Camano Island, and the North Cascades. The sun is still up (the sun sets close to ten at the height of summer). There are pleasure boats in the distance and people ambling along First Street, maybe hanging on the railing of the Boy and Dog Park, named for lifelike bronze statues by our local artist Georgia Gerber. Now that you are in the mood, maybe salivating a bit for the scene as well as the coming meal . . .

◈

Chef Sibrand Jurriaans Brussels Sprouts

Here's his narrative about the recipe:

I thought I'd share a simple recipe but one that means a lot to me. I used to hate Brussels sprouts, always overcooked and nasty until one night I ate them at a restaurant in Seattle: The Harvest Vine. They were crispy, sweet, spicy, and nothing like the mushy ones I remembered from my childhood. I fell in love with an ingredient I used to despise. When we opened Prima Bistro it was something I wanted to replicate so I set out to create my version of Brussels sprouts. What we do is trim the outer leaves, cut them in half, and blanch them first in very salty boiling water; a chef I once worked for told me that the water you blanch your vegetables in should be salty like the sea. They should blanch only for about 2 to 3 minutes, depending on the size; you want them to still be crunchy inside. We then cool them down in ice water to stop the cooking. For service we cook and serve them in little cast-iron skillets. Depending on the size of the pan you use, you want to melt down enough butter over high heat so that there is at least ⅛ inch of melted butter in the pan—you can always drain some out before you serve. Believe me, butter is the key. We then place our cut sprouts flat side down in the foaming butter until they get a nice golden brown color; like other cabbages they have a good amount of sugar, so the browning gives them a nice nutty flavor. We then add chopped garlic and fine herbs (tarragon, chives, fennel fronds, parsley), salt, and pepper, and they are ready to go. They are slightly crunchy, sweet, nutty, garlicky, and the richness of butter tops it off—delicious. Since we began the dish we have started doing business with Georgie from Willowood Farm, and her Brussels sprouts business has grown with our need. In the wine world they talk about "terroir," or "a sense of place"; this describes the essence of flavor in wine that occurs from where it is grown. I believe this is also true in the food world. The local produce we use speaks of the place it is grown and our Brussels sprouts are a sterling example.

Squash Bisque by Jess Dowdell

4 leeks

1 carrot

1 whole celery stalk

1 onion

¼ cup roughly chopped garlic (3–4 cloves)

2 tablespoons local butter or canola oil

1½ gallons vegetable stock

2 cups apple juice

1 gallon cooked squash from 1 large pumpkin, roasted

4 green apples, cored and chopped

¼ cup fresh minced ginger

⅛ cup chopped fresh sage

Salt and pepper to taste

Optional: cinnamon, allspice, and lemon

Roughly chop the leeks, carrot, celery, onion, and garlic and sauté together in a large pot in the local butter, about 5 to 8 minutes, until the onions are translucent. Add the stock and apple juice and cook on medium heat until the carrots are soft. Add the cooked squash insides, chopped apples, ginger, and sage. Cook for 15 minutes more or until the apples are just soft, then puree with a food processor. Add salt and pepper to taste. You can also add some cinnamon, allspice, and lemon to punch it up a little.

CHAPTER NINE

Bringing Our Eating Closer to Home

Stand still. The trees ahead and bushes beside you
Are not lost. Wherever you are is called Here
—David Wagoner

By the time February arrived local eating was a big ho-hum. After all
that preparation, the 50-mile diet was such a cinch that it was barely
worth writing about. After all, how long can anyone (but a food
writer) pay attention to the hundred or so times a day that food cycles
from the fridge to stove to plate to mouth to gut to, well, you get the
drift. I kept my new network of local food sources. My garden wound
down, but its hearty kale stuck with me through the winter. Molly's
CSA winter extender kept me in greens, tubers, and squash. I was
well stocked with flour, cabbage, roots, and hearty greens from Nash's
Farm in Sequim, beans from Georgie, grains from Lauren and Georgina, onions and squash from Tricia, plus gleaned apples and jars of
Belinda's tough old birds. More and more exotics crept in, sure, but I
now preferred relational eating to anywhere eating.

As I mentioned in the introduction, a new behavior, they say,
takes three weeks to go from conscious effort to established habit, at
which point it recedes into the background of "just what I do." Local
was now a habit. Good for me, but so what? It was an important first
step in change, but for me, that wasn't enough. I needed to understand how something so natural—eating where you live—became so
heroic, and how we can get back to the garden, so to speak, reinte-
grating food production into our communities.

261

Now I was chewing on the question, What if everyone did it?

As I'd learned even before beginning my diet, if everyone did it we'd quickly strip Whidbey of food. Even if just half of 1 percent of us ate exclusively from the island, we would use up all the local supplies. For example, a local mom-and-pop-type restaurant near me, Neil's Clover Patch, got the local-food bee in their bonnet and now buys hamburger from the Long Family Farm. Half of what they produce now goes to the restaurant, and we don't yet have a way to ramp up local beef production to meet the increased demand. Good news for Long's. A steady single market. Bad news for the rest of us. Competition for limited supply.

I hadn't planned to prove anything by my hyperlocal diet—except perhaps that I can do anything for a month. It was just going to be an adventure. Even after all my discoveries, I wasn't planning to march forward with a message for the world, once again donning my former lifestyle evangelist persona. I might have deflected these "How can everyone do it?" niggles and defaulted to a cheerful skepticism, but two things happened that kept me on the hunt for answers to bigger questions than "Where's my crunch?": a book and a dream.

The Book

Toward the end of September, as I found myself blogging that I was transforming my relationship with food the way I'd transformed my relationship with money, I had that wisp of a thought, I wonder if there is a book in here. I sent a link to that post to my *Your Money or Your Life* agent. She wrote right back, "Get me a proposal as soon as possible."

And so it was that as easily as a dizzy-in-love couple can forget protection and find themselves parents, I wrote the proposal, Beth sold it to my *Your Money or Your Life* publisher, Viking Penguin, and the seed of this book started to grow, reorganizing my life the way a fetus captures a mother's energy.

The Dream

The second event, a Technicolor dream, came two months after I was eating nuts and chocolate again. It was my first night in Brazil, where I was about to lead a tour. I was sleeping on the pullout sofa in my young Brazilian friend Thomas's small apartment in the hip Vila Madalena neighborhood of São Paulo.

In the dream Thomas was flying an old prop plane and I was somehow sitting on the nose in front of the propeller, relishing the wind, the sun, and the green landscape below. Then I slipped off, landing in a grassy field, surprisingly without hurting myself. I began to walk toward the horizon, waving to Thomas saying, "It's okay. I know my way home. I'll walk."

"No, you won't," he said, and, tipping the wing of the plane, he reached out his hand, grabbed me by the wrist, and up we went again, me swinging free, unafraid, relishing once more the air and light and landscape. But I was slipping.

"I can't hold on," I said and fell again, onto the field as lush as a golf course. "It's okay, I know my way home. I'll walk."

"No, you won't," he said again, tipping the wing, grabbing me, rising, and then tipping the plane in the other direction so my body draped over the nose and I could hoist myself up to straddle it again as I had before, in the air and light and freedom.

It wasn't hard for me to decode the dream. When I was in the grip of cancer, I "rehearsed" dying in long meditations. I know it can be, if we stay calm, a "going home," a liberation into spirit. In the dream I was quite happy to literally go "over the hill," off into the sunset, home. But clearly this young man—and his band of young creative-change agents—was having none of it. He/they wanted me to fly with them. Not as the crew, but as the figurehead on their ship. I had more work to do in partnership with the next generations. My time of retreat initiated by the cancer was over, almost seven years after it had begun.

Hope

Come, come, whoever you are.
Wanderer, worshipper, lover of leaving—it doesn't matter,
Ours is not a caravan of despair.
Come, even if you have broken your vow a hundred times,
Come, come again, come.[1]

As often happens with assignments that come in dreams, this one asked more of me than I had. Yet. If I was going to inspire, energize, fuel the dreams of the next generations, I needed more hope than I had. I'd gotten from despair to acceptance to cheerful adaptation through the idea of relocalization, but that was hardly a clarion call for young warriors. Welcome to a diminished world. Here's the mess we've made. Get busy, see what you can cobble together from it.

I hadn't actually lost hope. I'd buried it. I'd said a requiem for the planet at the turn of the millennium and poured a solid concrete slab over that crazy idea that we can stop the runaway train.

Against my better judgment, though, reason for hope was sprouting right between the cracks. My 10-mile diet had done far more than convince me that my island could be a sturdy locker of survival rations in the face of the triple crisis. Each day of the diet I learned more about our tainted food and denatured food systems—reason enough to lose hope again . . . but I didn't—because I was also becoming part of a growing community. In one sense, this means I was one of the people growing food and eating food grown locally. I was belonging. In another, I had stumbled into a widespread community of people working toward healthy food systems. In their company, it became natural to hope again.

Natural Hope

Hope is like fertility in the sense Chris Korrow, my biodynamic farmer, explained to me. It's not something we put into life; it comes out of life naturally, like warmth or a sweet smell. Our task is not to forcibly change bad situations but rather to notice the seeds of hope we might cultivate. We don't make hope. We cooperate with it.

This kind of hope isn't made by the will nor does it descend like grace from heaven. It isn't invented or imagined. It doesn't require proof or respond to moods. It's there all the time. It simply requires watering.

Nothing lives without hope, because hope is actually what every living thing expresses by getting up in the morning. Life hopes! Every second we're alive, hope is there in our steadily beating hearts and our breathing. Hope is as much a fact of life as babies—which are themselves evidence of life's hopeful tendencies.

I spent a few months volunteering at a hospice facility to prepare myself as best as I could for the imminent death of my partner, Joe Dominguez. I'd been shielded, as most of us have, from seeing people sicken and die, and I needed to participate in that process somehow. There at that hospice wing of a hospital I saw how the heart keeps hanging on to life even when the mind has surrendered or given up. I've seen people ready to die, wishing to die, who live on because life wants to take the next breath. Life goes on naturally.

"Life goes on" is not a weary statement of monotony, like Macbeth's "Tomorrow and tomorrow and tomorrow creeps in this petty pace from day to day."

"Life goes on" has the exuberant, inevitable power of a great waterfall.

Once I discovered this natural hope, it was easy to embrace it not as an antidote to the data but as a deeper truth in which the data is generated. The data doesn't contradict hope. Hope itself generates the data; why would researchers develop the data if not hoping to contribute to maintaining or improving life? If the data is disturbing, that's life at work, providing us with the kick in the pants we need to change. It worked with the ozone hole. Data showed up and we acted and the hole diminished. The weight of data is now pushing against policy makers, moving them (some would say glacially) toward climate remediation.

But honestly, there wasn't much reason for hope in the human world. Forests may regenerate, life may go on, but many think it has a better shot without our human presence.

In my new role as elder-on-a-nose-cone, do I just need to avoid the touchy subject of overshoot and collapse?

My breakthrough came when I realized I actually don't know what's going to happen a week from now, so how can I be sure that my predictions for a decade from now will be true. It's like seeing a car going south at sixty miles per hour on 525, Whidbey Island's backbone highway, and saying, as it passes you standing in Bayview, "That fella will drive right into Puget Sound in ten minutes." We might predict that, except we don't know if he'll slow down, turn onto a side road, get a flat tire, remember he left his wallet on the dresser and turn around, or get a speeding ticket. And we are certainly discounting that he'll probably drive onto a ferry and not simply sail off the pier.

The present suggests but doesn't predict because we can't see all the factors in play. A lot can change between a measurement and an outcome.

Saying you don't know how things will turn out doesn't deny the data, but it does allow you to release your convictions, widen your frame, see more options, head in a better direction, or slow down. As you do this, you might just find more hope-filled possibilities and turn your attention there.

I'd based my life for several decades on this overshoot data. I don't have to stop believing in it, ignoring everything the climate and resource scientists have said and the world's best minds have confirmed. I simply need to allow for some mystery and humility between today and fifty years from now.

As I was writing these words, news came that a mentor and friend for nearly thirty years passed away: Ernest "Chick" Callenbach, author of *Ecotopia* and wise elder of sane living. He composed a final essay as cancer was doing its dirty work, and tucked it into his hard drive to be opened after he was gone. Among the many wise ideas was this section on hope:

Hope. Children exude hope, even under the most terrible conditions, and that must inspire us as our conditions get worse. Hopeful patients recover better. Hopeful test candidates score better. Hopeful builders construct better buildings. Hopeful parents produce secure and resilient children. In groups, an atmosphere of hope is essential to shared successful effort: "Yes, we can!" is not an empty slogan, but a mantra for people who intend to do something together—whether it is rescuing victims of hurricanes, rebuilding flood-damaged buildings on higher ground, helping wounded people through first aid, or inventing new social structures (perhaps one in which only people are "persons," not corporations). We cannot know what threats we will face. But ingenuity against adversity is one of our species' built-in resources. We cope, and faith in our coping capacity is perhaps our biggest resource of all.

Understanding that even if my facts are correct my interpretations are not certainties liberated me to hope in a very new and invigorating way. I don't know how things will turn out. I don't know if what I'm doing will make much of a difference. But I know that life hopes, and if I choose to hope, to stand in hope, to BE hope, then I am headed where life naturally wants to go. Not only did this open me again to life—it seemed to my strategic mind like a winning strategy. Better to be a swivel-hipped quarterback looking for openings than a soldier with marching orders.

This felt like shaking off a dream. Or blinking into the daylight after being in a long tunnel. It felt like someone had snipped the string pinning my wings to my body so I could soar again. It felt, in short, like me. I was on the nose of that plane in the wind, with younger hands now on the controls. I was done resisting our slide into overshoot and collapse. My new assignment was to nourish life. Somehow.

Local Everywhere?

What better way to nourish life than relational eating! It's a daily act. What we eat is one way we vote on the future—a mouthful at a time. Also, buying local "buys" more local food capacity, which increases food security, soil fertility, and local prosperity. So I asked myself how my 10-mile experiment might have value for more than just me and my farmers and a few other people crazy enough to try it. Can local be one of those positive options that actually alters the outcome?

I like heading into the unknown with a powerful question so I asked, Can local really scale up to feed the people?

At first blush, scaling up local sounds ridiculous. You can't have large-scale small-scale. Local by its very nature is diverse, entrepreneurial, adaptive to microclimates, individualistic unto quirky. Local is relational.

Organic could scale up because it's about standards for growing food—seeds, practices, and inputs. There can be "organic everywhere," but local everywhere seems a contradiction in terms.

Do you scale up eaters? Increase the proportion of local for each eater in a locale? Increase the number of locavores, full converts, in a locale? Aim at 50 percent of your eaters on a 50/50 diet year-round?

Do you scale up farms? More cows for the Long family or more garlic from Georgie? Is that asking inherently small-scale family farms to grow beyond their natural lands, acquire more property, become an ever more vertically integrated business. Would "Long's beef" or "Georgie's garlic" become rootless brands, product pulled from anywhere. Cascadian Farms did that—grew beyond Gene Kahn's original berry patch and became a powerful brand. In doing so, it left the community behind—the berries came from everywhere—though not the values.

Do you scale up land in production, get new farmers onto fallow land so that we double, triple, or more the number of five-acre-and-under properties in production? More farmers on fallow land would increase farm stands, CSAs, farmers' markets, supplies for grocers and restaurants. That's closer, but if these new farmers are going to fare well financially, they need a system of financial fairness, not just a few customers who can afford to pay the true cost.

I sat with these contradictions until the next key insight showed up. I realized I had stumbled into a rigged fight. How can local win in a contest for who will feed the world? If "scale up" means to get big enough to pump food out to the masses, it's guaranteed that local would lose.

"Put everyone on a local diet," the industrial system says through its many mouthpieces, "and people would starve. Civilizations would collapse. We'd be back in the Dark Ages, serfs with hoes. With seven billion people on the planet, there is no alternative to the food industrial complex."

There is no alternative. Where had I heard that before? Ah, a dozen years earlier when Margaret Thatcher, speaking for neoliberal economic policies, said TINA—there is no alternative—to corporate globalization. What global civil society said on the streets of Seattle in 1999, protesting the WTO (World Trade Organization), and in every year since, was "There are many alternatives! And we are living them now!"

Maybe local can't feed the world the way the global industrial system does, but "locals feeding locals" can multiply sideways, linking arms. In fact, this is already happening. The strength of local is the very everywhere-ness of it, the guerrilla-ness of it.

Now we are on new ground with a new question. How can local scale sideways—and feed the world? I like that question. In it I see the hope I've been seeking, a place to stand, actions to take, and a humble attitude. No longer fixated on fixing or stopping things, I can participate in restoring, regenerating, and relocalizing life. You could call it "relational hope." In fact, I think I will.

It Takes a System to Feed a Village

If vertical integration is the key strategy of global brands, then horizontal distribution with webs of relationships is the strategy of scaling local sideways. We need to repair our food web. We need a system to support all the people and institutions that bring local food to our table: the growers, distributors, butchers, packagers, processors, marketers, retail outlets, chefs, lenders, advocates, educators, and artists. It takes a system to feed a village, to paraphrase the old African proverb.

Local food scales neighbor to neighbor, network to network, relational every step of the way, putting trust and community first. We can see that clearly in farmers' markets. The market itself is a technology for connecting growers to the public and to one another such that everyone wins. We can see that through Mike Nichols of Whidbey Green Goods, who increases local production by encouraging small growers to grow a bit more for market—and then sells their food to his customers. We see it at Grange meetings and at county fairs, those once-a-year extravaganzas for the food, farming, animal husbandry, processing, educational, and commerce communities to strut their stuff, dance, gossip, and meet and greet.

The USDA's definition of local as four hundred miles—as silly as that seems to hyperlocavores—actually helps us imagine "local everywhere." Four hundred miles delineates a region, not just a city or even county. True regional agriculture is defined more by geography and climate than by distance, yet at least this four-hundred-mile local opens up that space of relational hope. We can link up and strengthen regional food systems so that appropriately-sized farms, stores, distributors, and processing plants can flourish together, leapfrogging from one success to the next.

Could such regional food and farming networks supply even 10 percent, or a bodacious 25 percent, or a miraculous 50 percent, of what their eaters need to survive? Could each of us stand in the middle of where we live, as I was learning to do, and look out on a flourishing landscape of food as far as the eye could see? In cities we'd see yards and rooftops and community gardens. Farther we'd see farmland and dairies and ranches oriented around feeding their region. Farther we'd of course see larger-scale operations with a global reach, hopefully with fair wages and good working conditions and healthy practices and good corporate citizenship. Farther still (if you live in a temperate climate) you'd see the tropics, with coffee, tea, fruit, and spices, grown sustainably and traded fairly.

Take a moment now and look out from where you live to the landscapes of food, the windowsill, the yard, the neighborhood, city, region, nation, and communities around the world. See food everywhere—all of it relational, as in knowable by you. Now imagine someone a thousand miles away likewise standing and looking out on his or her food system, eventually overlapping with yours. Imagine everyone everywhere being able to stand in food systems that feed their people and feed their hope.

A Local World

To do this exercise for myself, I simply got out my map and ruler. The 50-miles-as-the-crow-flies diet I undertook in February got me south almost to Olympia, north almost to Bellingham, west out to Sequim on the Olympic Peninsula, where Nash's large market garden is, and east to the foothills of the Cascade Mountains. This is, in fact, Puget Sound, a natural basin that nourished the Coast Salish tribes for millennia and the early settlers of the region for a century plus. One hundred miles, a more common measure for locavores, would reach over to the Yakima Valley to bring me ample warm-weather fruits and vegetables—tomatoes, peaches, apricots, grapes, peppers, as well as hops (yum, beer), oats, wheat, and barley—plus a lot more meat. A USDA "local," four hundred miles, would reach into Oregon, northern California, Idaho, and Montana and well into British Columbia, almost to Manitoba. Exploring these food ranges, I realized how well we would eat should we, by choice or necessity, confine ourselves to a four-hundred-mile radius.

Oh, yeah? you might say. What about New York City? Gotcha.

Out came the ruler and another map.

Ten miles was ridiculous. Measuring from Times Square, you'd get a bit west of the Jersey Turnpike, south to Coney Island, east to Bayside, Queens, and north to the Bronx and Yonkers. When my mother was born you'd find farmland in that circle. Not now. Even with the advent of gardens and chicken coops on rooftops—and CSA gardens in the city limits—these are barely pinholes of hope. But when you look at that USDA four-hundred-mile range, hope seems less like a dream and more like reality. As the crow flies, you could get to Detroit or Raleigh or Quebec from Manhattan, with thousands of acres of beautiful farmland in every direction.

Food 2020

I decided to start testing this notion of "local everywhere" by investigating my own Whidbey Island food system, then fanning out to the hundred-mile six-county region. What is growing, in terms of food but also innovations, within this circle? How can I, a lowly eater, contribute to creating a dense, rich food web here?

Fortunately, a Transition Whidbey action group had produced a comprehensive food system report several years earlier (see box below).

MAPPING YOUR SYSTEM

If you want to change a system, you have to start with where you are. In systems thinking, you need to measure "stocks" (what you have) and "flows" (what passes through your system, and the route it takes). If you want to lose weight, you get on the scale to see where you are, moderate or measure what you eat, get on the scale again, adjust diet and exercise, and eventually lose the intended weight . . . or not.

Same with a food system. You can say, "We want more local food in our stores," but until you understand the system, your work will be piecemeal, improvisational, and may not produce the change you seek.

On Whidbey our Transition group produced a food system report. They began the report saying, "A food systems 'map' is more than a visual list of who is growing what and where. It is a description of the larger loop of food production, harvesting, processing, distribution, and consumption that involves us all. It is a tool useful for increasing our awareness of the components of our food system (including its gaps and overlaps), better positioning us to engage in making the system increasingly resilient and sustainable."

Drawing on reports, government data, and other sources, they documented

- the top state, regional, and local food crops
- the various organizations promoting local food
- our ag resources: land zoned for agriculture, soil qualities, forests, seashore
- wild-food harvest: hunting, fishing, foraging
- the number of large and small farms
- farmland acres by crop

Analyzing the data, they identified gaps:

- While Island County generates more than $335,000 in livestock revenue, we have no meat-processing capability.
- While we generate more than $2 million in sales of fruits and vegetables, much flows off the island into the commodity markets. We have few commercial kitchens.
- While we have several farmers' markets, direct sales cost the farmers time off the farm. We have little local food in the markets.
- While more and more eaters want local food, until a farmer can guarantee a market or menu a consistent ample supply of standard, the buyers don't have time to manage relationships with many farmers and don't want to lose customers because standard fare is not available.
- Another supply-chain gap is the time, gas, and risk for farmers to become local delivery people.

But, they said, none of these gaps and challenges is insurmountable. It is possible!

Food system asset mapping can start with simple satisfaction surveys and go on to more complex focus groups and data-mining efforts to get a clear snapshot of the state of the systems.

An online community food satisfaction survey can be sent out widely. You can ask:

- How satisfied are you with the availability of local food in this community?
- How satisfied are you with the quantity of local food?
- How satisfied are you with the quality of local food?
- How much more are you willing to pay for local food over industrial food?
- What's in the way of you buying and using local food?
  — Price
  — Availability
  — Don't know how to cook it
  — Not convenient to buy it
  — Not used to it in my menus
  — Don't like it
  — Other
- What local food would you like more of, all things being equal?
- If you buy local food, where do you go to buy it?

More and more communities are far more systematic in their approach.

The Center for Whole Communities inspired a dedicated group of citizens and professionals to develop the Whole Measures for Community Food Systems, which is a mapping tool for the following comprehensive factors:

Justice and Fairness

- Provides food for all
- Reveals, challenges, and dismantles injustice in the food system

- Creates just food system structures and cares for food system workers
- Ensures that public institutions and local businesses support a just community food system

Strong Communities

- Improves equity and responds to community food needs
- Contributes to healthy neighborhoods
- Builds diverse and collaborative relationships, trust, and reciprocity
- Supports civic participation, political empowerment, and local leadership

Vibrant Farms

- Supports local, sustainable family farms to thrive and be economically viable
- Protects and cares for farmers and farmworkers
- Honors stories of food and farm legacy through community voices
- Respects farm animals

Healthy People

- Provides healthy food for all
- Ensures the health and well-being of all people, inclusive of race and class
- Connects people and the food system, from field to fork
- Connects people and land to promote health and wellness

Sustainable Ecosystems

- Sustains and grows a healthy environment
- Promotes an ecological ethic
- Enhances biodiversity
- Promotes agricultural and food distribution practices that mitigate climate change

Thriving Local Economies

- Creates local jobs and builds long-term economic vitality within the food system
- Builds local wealth
- Promotes sustainable development while strengthening local food systems
- Includes infrastructure that supports community and environmental health.[2]

This led me on a fascinating journey to conversations with old friends and new and to a meeting with more than fifty people involved in the food system on Whidbey. With each conversation I got more clues—and discovered more roadblocks. This next section takes you on this hunt with me—and points to reasonable, actionable hope that, as relational eaters, you and I can steer our ship of food toward flourishing regional food systems.

Being relational to the core, my first stop on the research train would be to find the local experts. Next stop—since I believe that all serious change begins in conversation among people who care—would be to set up what's called a "multistakeholder dialogue." For that I needed my experts to identify the stakeholders, the members of my Whidbey food system—the farmers, ranchers, foodies, gardeners, marketers, activists, purchasing agents, educators, and more.

Providentially, right about then I sat down with Maryon Attwood, by vocation a potter, by profession working to integrate the Whidbey food system, and by instinct a practical visionary whose key talent is her ability to create systems out of loose networks, to get a hodgepodge of individuals into mutually beneficial alliances.

When I first met her, Maryon was working for the Northwest Agricultural Business Center, a nonprofit seeking to increase profits for agricultural businesses—farmers, distributors, processors, and markets. She helped develop the Whidbey Grown brand to distinguish our local producers in a competitive marketplace. Maryon's patient systems work impressed me. She later helped get the Greenbank Farm New Farmer Training Center off the ground. This program trains half a dozen young people a year in the whole spectrum of farming skills, from planting to marketing to writing a business plan.

When I began thinking and writing about the food system, I turned to Maryon to give me the lay of the land, so to speak. We hitched ourselves up on the bar stools at my kitchen counter, wrapped our hands around cups of hot tea, and got to know each other. When I tendered my idea of getting the whole food and farming system in a room for a day for a "Can we feed ourselves?" conversation, Maryon said the magic words: "Let's do it." I had a partner in relational hope.

We put out the call to our networks for help. The perfect planning team assembled effortlessly.

Judy Feldman at that time ran the Washington State University/ Island County 4-H program, though she has since moved on to becoming executive director of the nonprofit Greenbank Farm.

Karen Lazarus, a professor at Antioch University in Seattle, had cowritten, with Judy, Maryon, and two others, a report, *Exploring Island County's Food System,* which became my research bible. They'd started out to do an apparently simple job—identify all the growers on the island and put them on a map for all to see. As they ferreted out farmers, though, they realized these individuals were part of an as yet unmapped food system—the soils, crops, history, and laws as well as the farms, farmers, and crops. If we are to feed ourselves from here, we need to know what actually *is* here.

Jean Singer also taught at Antioch and brought two other key pieces to the table. First, she is a professional facilitator (as is Karen). Second, she and her partner, Dyanne, are members of a social group in Maxwelton Valley that evolved into a micro food cooperative, with each member growing different crops to share with the group. They rarely need to go to the store during the growing half of the year.

Terra Anderson also has a goal of growing all her family's food on their ten acres, but as one dedicated gardener (plus husband with tractor).

Britt Conn joined the circle too; she and Eric, you will remember, have a farm where they grow for CSA customers and the farmers' market. She was at the time the coordinator of the Sustainable Whidbey Coalition.

Rhiannon Fisher committed to cooking all the food! When asked why she was so committed to sustainability she said, "I'm a mom." One of her many dreams is to do that asset map of the island, so Food 2020 was right up her alley.

Later I reflected on the composition of that group meeting in the back room of the South Whidbey Commons, a teen-run coffeehouse and bookstore. All of us were growers, some for ourselves, some for families, some for market. We were all tenders of community— educators, writers, facilitators, executive directors, moms. And we were all systems thinkers, people able to see how things link together, how everything is part of the whole.

We called our event Food 2020 and we posited the outrageous: that 50 percent of the food eaten on the island would be grown on the island by 2020.

Given how outlandish that goal was, it's a miracle that sixty busy, practical people involved in food and farming showed up. On a sunny day in May no less!

Jean and Karen designed the day, using several tools from their facilitation bag of tricks—moving people among small groups for conversations and gathering the whole group for discussion.

They asked me to seed the visioning part of the day with a brief meditation.

"It's 2020. Good morning. Open your eyes. Fifty percent of the food we eat here on Whidbey grows here. Look around. Where is food grown? What is grown? Who grows it? How does it get to market? What do we eat? How is the soil tended? Water? Waste? Kitchens? Restaurants? Processing? What do you see, smell, hear, taste, feel? Don't worry how we got here, just cruise around (bike, foot, car, golf cart—anything works) and marvel."

After ten minutes of silence, we huddled in small groups and talked about what we'd imagined. We each scribbled specific visions on Post-its. We then gathered at a wall covered with butcher paper, put up our Post-its, arranged the ideas in patterns, and stepped back to marvel at our shared vision of the future.

Here's a snapshot.

The grocery stores up and down the island are all hybrids, plenty of industrial food but so much locally grown food you'd think they were co-ops: meats, vegetables, and fruits, plus staples like grains, beans, and flour, plus foraged foods like chanterelles and nettles, plus canned and bottled foods like sauces, wines, jellies, soups, honey. Given the rise in the prices of oil and gas, prices for local foods are finally competitive. You can swing by any farm to buy fresh veggies at their self-serve stand—but backyard gardeners also set out their excess for purchase. Micro food networks have formed among neighbors who together plan what each will grow—and share. Restaurants focus their menus on what's fresh—or what is stored over winter. Whidbey is a culinary tourism destination, with solar-powered tour buses meeting the ferries for a series of gastronomic and educational adventures.

In addition to home delivery systems, we have two food hubs, north and south. Trucks fan out every day, picking up produce from farms, bringing it to the hub, putting together orders to stock the restaurants and grocers, as well as filling orders from the hospital, schools, and the naval air station. Each hub has a retail section where people can buy fresh food and enjoy a soup and bread lunch (the bread made from fresh-milled local flour leavened by sourdough starter from our free-range wild yeast spores and lactic-acid bacteria).

The big box stores all carry local food too—Walmart, Safeway. In fact, in 2020 Walmart sponsors three young farmers a year at the Greenbank Farm New Farmer Training Center and has partnered with WILC—Whidbey Island Local Compost—giving them all their discarded produce.

All the schools have their own gardens, run by students and forming the basis of school lunches. The hospital actually has its own farm and farmer to provide healthy greens daily.

Indeed, food is everywhere. We bring potluck dishes to most events—performances, lectures, church, fund-raisers, and dances. Everyone eats and no one goes hungry (a goal we were already reaching in 2011 through our web of caring organizations). We are food-prosperous (which actually means hopeful!), with jobs in agriculture, food service, farm and garden supplies, and related industries supporting island families. Banks, investment groups, and small-time lenders have all opened the faucet of financial support for many dozens of food and farming businesses.

Not only is there no hunger but people appreciate every bite—and take fewer of them. Food is more precious because it's overall more expensive—and the local food is grown by people we know. As happened in Cuba after Russia withdrew its oil shipments, we are all thinner and more able. In fact, we are sick less and treat most illnesses with patience, rest, and locally formulated tonics, infusions, roots, and leaves—though we also still rely on surgery and antibiotics as needed. Some farms grow medicinal plants exclusively.

With oil now tripled in price, we produce more energy locally from the sun, winds, tides, and biomass (including poop), but it's pricey too, so some have returned to animal power—oxen and horses—to run their farms. With demand for locally grown food soaring, more five- to ten-acre farms are actively using permaculture, biodynamic, organic, and agro-ecological strategies to grow food intensively. Farming itself is no longer a marginal profession since the economics of the global food system have shifted due to declining fertility, changing weather patterns, and rising energy costs. It's just more cost-effective to source food regionally.

Some hobby farmers have given up their city homes and moved here lock, stock, and (rain) barrel. Tax breaks for putting at least 50 percent of their property in agriculture encouraged some of them to even give five-year leases to young farmers who grow food for them and the community. All this means the average age of farmers on Whidbey is now under fifty, and the longtime farmers find themselves in demand as educators and mentors to flocks of people in their twenties eager to learn farming and grow food. The Greenbank Farm New Farmer Training Center now graduates fifty farmers a year and Skagit Valley College has a certificate program in organic farming as well. Most farms have a seed-saving program, cultivating seeds that flourish in our microclimates. Besides Walmart waste, WILC converts all island organic waste into good soil. In fact, composting toilets are now legal as third bathrooms.

Bottom line: In 2020 we now have the capacity to provide one thousand calories a day of nutritious, delicious, seasonal food for all our people—who, by the way, have learned to design their daily menus around what we can produce.

The next step after visioning was "back casting"—standing in that 2020 vision and telling the story, year by year, of how we got here from 2011. That was harder. Our doubting, discouraged minds spoke up then: Impossible! They won't let us! We don't have the money! Who will do it?

I gave folks three ". . . and then a miracle happened" cards so they could think in terms of possibility rather than drudgery. Even so, when we put our ideas on a time line and contemplated the work before us, many felt anticipatory exhaustion—and slowly filtered out of the building, saying their gardens were calling.

By three P.M., when it was time to form working groups, 60 percent of the participants were gone. Still, three groups formed: farmer cooperatives, finance mechanisms for farming, and establishing a multistakeholder food policy council.

And then . . . nothing happened. Apparently. But that is from the point of view of the industrial food system.

Now, two years after this meeting when "nothing really happened," I can see many new shoots and swelling buds of projects—a grain cooperative, a composting business, and more. W.I.L.L. is up and running with more than $200,000 in individual loans made so far. A grant has come through for a commercial kitchen at the county fairground. Several more restaurants now serve local menus. Two new farmers' markets opened, a new sheep-milk dairy is licensed, a farmer bought dry-pack equipment to package her lavender, a conference on thriving communities focused on food drew people from across the region. An alliance between Good Cheer Food Bank and several other organizations, called Fresh Food for the Table, has begun paying a young farming couple to grow vegetables for the food bank all year long. CSAs are multiplying.

I believe that the Food 2020 exercise fed our imaginations, gave us hope, seeded alliances and friendships, and created a mental map we each carry about how the people who live here can live from here. We are moving not like an organization but like an ecosystem. That speaks of wisdom. We are cultivating, not manufacturing, a local food future.

You could say, "Oh, it was just a few Post-its. Most people left, having better things to do on a sunny afternoon in May." Or you can understand that we could now see our food system working, and see seeds in action.

HOW TO DO A FOOD 2020 EVENT

Food 2020 is what we called our food system visioning and community mobilizing event. There are many approaches to community organizing and participatory planning, so rather than a recipe I'll give you key ingredients.

Develop a core team, making sure each member has a real interest in the prosperity of your farms, farmers, ranchers, and all the systems that bring food to the table. Be sure to invite some key players already working "in the field," so to speak: agency and NGO representatives. Agree on a motivating purpose for your event.

Make a guest list of everyone involved in the food system in your locale. Include in your brainstorming produce and grain farmers (from CSA growers to field crop farmers), livestock farmers, dairy(wo)men, grocers, farmers' markets, institutional purchasers (hospitals, schools, churches, feeding programs), advocacy groups, elected officials, distributors, educators (farmer training, teachers), grant makers, lenders . . . oh, yes, and eaters who care!

Engage one or two really good facilitators (volunteer or paid) who have familiarity with the techniques you'll use. I use, as needed, open space, World Café, Conversation Café, dynamic facilitation, TOP (technology of participation) processes, and comedy improv. Whatever keeps the group creative, focused, moving forward. A graphic facilitator helps keep the group focused and produces a beautiful picture of the essence of what is said. This picture is a record and can be unfurled at future meetings for inspiration.

Pick a date and a big room with movable chairs.

Craft an invitation. Here's the one we sent for our May 2011 event:

We hope you can join us for a special daylong event on May 23, 2011, called Food 2020. We'll meet at 9:30 at the Unitarian Church north of Freeland and spend the day visioning and planning for a more vital and prosperous food system on Whidbey.

In the last three years there has been an explosion of activity supporting local food on Whidbey Island. Today, we have a real opportunity to rehabilitate our whole local food system for the people who live and work on Whidbey Island.

What would a thriving local food system look like in 2020? One that could produce, process, and deliver half of the food we eat each year. Once Whidbey had a bountiful food system, sufficient for the basic needs of those who lived here. With "local food" now as popular as "organic food"—and with our assets of climate, seashore, soils, and farmers—it can benefit every one of us to work together toward reclaiming this bounty.

Many cities and counties across the United States—and world—are reorienting their food systems to provide a greater percentage of daily needs locally. It's called "food sovereignty and security." Local not only means fresh food for citizens and economic prosperity for farmers. It also means greater autonomy and sustainability.

Whidbey Island is certainly one of those special places that can achieve what so many want: healthy, fresh food grown and sold closer to home.

The first step is to bring together the local capital that abounds on Whidbey Island. That's you and other local citizens. The power of the community and the chance for achievable final goals resides in people like you—involved in the activities, in the thinking, in the work.

We recognize that a full day in the spring is a very valuable resource, and we promise you an excellent day on every level: informative, useful, and enjoyable—with a delicious lunch, great networking, and the promise of clarity about actions that will help all of us prosper. Your perspective is important, as invitees represent a balance of players in our food system. We value the wisdom and experience you bring.

We also know that rehabilitating our local food system is a considerable challenge. That is why we need a day to step back and look at the big picture and develop a vision of prosperity and vitality to inspire us to do the work to get there.

Our event included a short guided meditation inviting participants to wake up in 2020 to 50 percent of our food sourced locally—and smell the herbal tea, the breakfast cooking, to walk around, observe food growing and being sold and eaten. Then we did a World Café, where people fleshed out this vision in three successive groups of four. We then did a brainstorm where we harvested the features people saw of our 2020 system. After a yummy local lunch we did a "back casting" process in which we imagined standing in our 2020 vision and talked about the sequence of events that happened to get us there. Finally, we had an open space to form action groups.

At the end of your event, celebrate your guests and the day . . . and go home and see what happens.

On a neighboring island, Orcas, a group has hosted a Food Charrette. Rhea Miller, the spark plug for the event, sent me her description of it in an e-mail:

Set a format to inspire, inform, and incite action for increasing access to healthy, local food. Form a small group of interested stakeholders ahead of time, to determine what windows of opportunity are presenting them-selves. These opportunities are translated into work groups for the char-rette. A winter day, often in February when folks are beginning to think about gardens again, is chosen for the charrette to ensure that farmers can be present. The day begins with inspiring video shorts, online food quizzes, and our community's story of food so far, always mindful that there may be people present who are new to the topic. Then the whole group self-selects into smaller work groups, at times using the Conversation Café pro-tocol. The first year the work groups focused on growing grain, supporting the school's Farm and Garden program, and assessing our local food shed. The second year there were groups focused on a community food process-ing center or commercial kitchen and addressing hunger in the community. The latest charrette addressed the need for a GMO-free county and the formation of a seed library/bank. A healthy lunch is provided for a small fee. The day closes with feedback to the larger group. One charrette addi-tionally closed with a plant and seed exchange, as well as desserts. Each charrette keeps in mind the needs of the local community.

Write a story or report based on the day. This becomes the property of each member of the group so new ideas and initiatives can be born of what is present.

Remember the unwelcome wisdom that "everything takes longer than you think it will" and trust that under the surface much is growing and bubbling.

Naturalist Paul Krapfel, in his small, self-published book, *Shifting,* describes an experience of sitting out a rainstorm in a cave. Trapped for quite a while, he had time to observe the drops aggregate into rivulets that formed little channels for the water to flow. Then he no-ticed that if he moved just a few grains of sand, the whole flood plain of rivulets shifted. He learned that while you can't stop the rain, you can redirect the flow. He wondered if such microshifts could actually heal a damaged landscape—like a parched, denuded vacant lot in Los Angeles deeply rutted by runoff. Rather than come in with bulldozers and seeds to make the lot green again, Krapfel observed the flow of water across this patch of land and, moving handfuls of sand here and there, fanned the water out, filling ruts, making hospitable nooks for passing seeds to root. Eventually the gullies were gone, the grass returned, and the lot had become a meadow, a living system.

This is how our change feels to me: that slowly, grain by grain, gain by gain, we are restoring our food system by working with our wealth of fertility in a spirit of natural hope.

Can we restore our regional food systems the way Krapfel restored that field? One practical visionary doing just that is my old friend Richard Conlin.

Seattle's Quiet Food Evolution

Richard is a longtime member of the Seattle City Council. Phyllis Shulman, also an old friend, is his right-hand person. It was easy to pick up the phone and make an appointment with them to find out how Seattle was moving intentionally toward a local food future. It turns out they are doing cutting-edge work in classic low-key Seattle style.

Richard and I met in 1990 at a Seattle multistakeholder sustainability dialogue—not much different from Food 2020—convened to explore the newly minted value of sustainable development. He arrived on a bicycle and was wearing bicycle shorts, a sweaty T-shirt, and a helmet. His curly hair, whipped sideways by the wind, made him look a bit like Clarabell the Clown, but his comments were so cogent, informed, and radical without being aggressive that it is no surprise that within a decade he was on the city council. His hair is now cropped and gray, and he's become an insider, but he's still radical and so congenial and well liked, he's been able to get a lot done.

In 2008 he and Phyllis established the Local Food Action Initiative to create goals and a policy framework, and to identify specific actions to strengthen Seattle and the region's food system in a sustainable and secure way.

Slowly, quietly, and incrementally, policies shifted. A goat ordinance let people own up to three miniature goats—as pets, lawnmowers, and dairy animals for milk and cheese. The P-Patch program expanded. Owning pot-bellied pigs became legal. Homeowners could legally use their parking strips (city property) to grow vegetables. Seattle wrote its own set of Farm Bill Principles.

SEATTLE FARM BILL PRINCIPLES

Supporting Healthy Farms, Food and People

Guidance for the 2012 Farm Bill

HEALTH-CENTERED FOOD SYSTEM

The driving principle of the Farm Bill must be the relationship of food and ecologically sound agriculture to public health. Food that promotes health includes fruits, vegetables, whole grains, nuts, seeds, legumes, dairy, and lean protein. Improving the health of the nation's residents must be a priority in developing policies, programs, and funding.

SUSTAINABLE AGRICULTURAL PRACTICES

Promote farming systems and agricultural techniques that prioritize the protection of the environment so that the soil, air, and water will be able to continue producing food long into the future. Integral to both domestic and global agricultural policies should be agricultural techniques and farming practices that enhance environmental quality, build soil and soil fertility, protect natural resources and ecosystem diversity, improve food safety, and increase the quality of life of communities, farmers and farm workers.

COMMUNITY AND REGIONAL PROSPERITY AND RESILIENCE

Enhance food security by strengthening the viability of small and mid-scale farms, and increasing appropriately scaled processing facilities, distribution networks, and direct marketing. Develop strategies that foster resiliency, local innovation, interdependence, and community development in both rural and urban economies. Opportunities that create fair wage jobs are key to a strong economy.

EQUITABLE ACCESS TO HEALTHY FOOD

Identify opportunities and reduce barriers by developing policies and programs that increase the availability of and improve the proximity of healthy, affordable, and culturally-relevant food to urban, suburban, and rural populations. Protect the nation's core programs that fight food insecurity and hunger while promoting vibrant, sustainable agriculture.

SOCIAL JUSTICE AND EQUITY

The policies reflected in the Farm Bill impact the lives and livelihoods of many people, both in the U.S. as well as abroad. Develop policies, programs, and strategies that support social justice, worker's rights, equal opportunity, and promote community self-reliance.

SYSTEMS APPROACH TO POLICY MAKING

It is essential to reduce compartmentalization of policies and programs, and to approach policy decisions by assessing their impact on all aspects of the food system including production, processing, distribution, marketing, consumption, and waste management. Consider the interrelated effects of policies and align expected outcomes to meet the goal of a comprehensive health-focused food system.[3]

Because implementation of our Food 2020 vision seemed painfully slow to me, I asked Phyllis to give me the lowdown on how and why Seattle had made so much progress toward being a city that farms.

We met at the Grateful Bread in Seattle, the very café where friends and I started our first Conversation Café in 2001 and launched a global movement. It was a fitting place for a conversation about system change.

Phyllis outlined their winding pathway to that food security initiative. In the beginning, it wasn't about food at all. It was about Katrina. Watching the chaos was enough to send chills up the spine of a city sitting on a fault due to deliver "the big one" any day. How would Seattle cope? Richard's office asked, "What is resilience for a city, and what can a government do to foster it?"

They discovered that food is a resilience issue everyone can agree on, so food would be their focus for their resilience work. Food security would help the city withstand emergency chaos. It also linked the largest number of issues and organizations. So they convened a Local Food Action Initiative.

Eventually Richard helped convene a King County Food Policy Council in his signature style—convening, listening, proposing, reporting, passing ordinances, and making small projects happen again and again and again. Their 2009 FARMS (Future of Agriculture Realizing Meaningful Solutions) Report presents the findings of a study determining what measures King County should take to assure a healthy food future. Skimming it, I found a chart called, simply, "How Much Land Is Needed to Feed King County's Population?" Not a page-turner by a long shot, but in terms of my Food 2020 quest it gave me shivers of hope. They identified twenty-eight fruits and vegetables that grow well in their region. They cataloged the agricultural land still farmable in the county. They calculated potential yields for each crop—and discovered that King County could be 100 percent food secure in terms of vegetables. They could grow enough for everyone.[4]

Please pause with me to say, "Wow." Pie in the sky just became pie on the plate—nice apple pie!

Now pause to consider their findings about meat. They calculated how much land might be needed to raise livestock for consumption. For each type of meat they calculated how much land would be needed to produce 100 percent of what is consumed in the county. For example, for beef it would take 372,000 acres to raise all the beef that county residents consume. Given that they have only six thousand acres, they could produce only 1 percent of what's needed. The same is true for all meats—except chicken!

They can supply 100 percent of their need for chicken because chickens cohabit gardens. Think chicken tractors—mobile coops to use chicken's natural scratching and pecking to till new garden plots. Think New York City, where people raise chickens on roofs for fresh eggs! Think a roast chicken, green peas, and potatoes along with that apple pie.

I suspect goats could cohabit yards as well, providing some meat, milk, and cheese. Think a bit of cheese beside that apple pie.

Think, "Hmm, what about where I live?"

Complementary Food Systems

Of course this is a report about potential. There's a lot of work to actualize the potential—in King County and in your four-hundred-mile "local" area.

Regional food systems won't replace the global industrial one anytime soon—if ever. My hunch, however, is that we can revitalize and rely on them, bit by bit, as complementary food systems. In medicine, as good science verified the efficacy of alternative treatments, such practices were sanctioned—and insured—under the rubric of "complementary medicine." The same could happen with food—a more integral way of feeding ourselves.

Richard and Phyllis began their food policy work through the door of community resilience—the ability to weather short-term emergencies. Restoring the vitality of regional food systems could be seen as a strategy for longer emergencies arising from climate, energy, or economic disruptions. We need backup systems that can grow into complementary systems. In Russia, after the Soviet Union collapsed, people who had dachas, plots of land in the country, grew food. In Cuba they'd mobilized for food production and survived. In Greece and Ireland, as their economies shrank, people with ties to families in the countryside were able to grow food. Heck, in the United States during World War II, 20 million Americans planted victory gardens, providing up to 40 percent of all the vegetables consumed nationally.[5]

Living with Less Meat

For those of us who believe that such changes are on the way—and are vegetarians—this King County food system report is extremely good news. We meat eaters, though, will need to eat less—especially less red meat—and only sustainably raised, pastured meat.

There are three ways to do this other than cold turkey, which of course is a very poor choice of metaphor.

• First is the sustainability-as-an-extreme-sport approach of "I can do anything for a month." Set a constraint on your meat eating and live within it for a month. At the end see what you honestly have learned and want to carry forward. As I've said, my meat constraint in my 10-mile diet was that it cost so darn much I halved consumption and doubled investigation of my assumptions about protein. Prior to the 10-mile diet, I averaged six to eight ounces of meat a day. Now I'm down to two to three. I eat meat as a treat— and it really is! I take pleasure in that first rush of meatness, but by a few bites I'm back on automatic, so why eat more?

• Second is the 10 percent trick. Eat 10 percent less. Then another 10 percent less. Keep going until you've gone too far. Anyone can imagine doing 10 percent more or 10 percent less of anything. You could easily eat 10 percent less meat by skipping meat one day a week (that would technically be 14 percent) or eat 10 percent smaller portions—six ounces instead of seven.

• Third is to raise your own meat. Keeping chickens—within limits—is legal in hundreds of cities in the United States, including New York. If you raise, slaughter, and butcher your own animals, you tend to honor that meat. At the rate I eat meat, a chicken a month would be sufficient—plus I'd get a few eggs a week. At the rate I travel, though, I can't keep animals, so I happily pay my neighbors for raising my meat and eggs.

• Of course there are others, like Meatless Monday (or whatever day you choose), mentioned earlier.

Hope—After All

The King County report is now part of what gives me hope. It is natural for our region to feed us. It can be done. Even though our way of life—our gadgets, our assumptions, our entitlements—might be severely compromised, "we"—the whole community of life—is not off the cliff. We are simply crossing a great divide, which we have done many times before as we've evolved for billions of years on this planet. I mourn the suffering, I mourn what is dying, but I am now free to participate in what is growing. Okay, so I'm not Moses, but this careful examination of our prospects has at least parted the Red Sea of despair in my own mind.

Serotiny

Anytime I feel that hope requires that hypermissionary zeal that exhausted me in the nineties, I ground myself . . . literally. I go into my yard and let life fill me. However paved the earth, however complex our lives, however large our problems, I take comfort and refuge in the fact that under the surface life is going about its business, waiting for the right conditions to send up a shoot and have at it again.

I saw this miracle in practice many times in my years on the road. I often camped in landscapes recently devastated by fire—yet carpeted in magenta fireweed, a plant designed to come alive when a forest is mowed down. The tall fireweed becomes the shelter where other seedlings, like lodgepole pines, can develop. The cones of a lodgepole pine are sealed tight with a resin that melts only in the heat of a fire, releasing the seed to begin "foresting" again. This "coming to life after fire" is a type of serotiny—delays in blooming until conditions are right.

These pines remind me that what is scarred is merely cleared. What is burned is nutrient for what comes next. The fireweed isn't the winner, but simply the herald of a succession of lives, the beginning of the next mature forest. In life, hope is hospitality—making a good bed where the next guest in the landscape can find shelter. This is how life always behaves.

From the point of view of the forest, cities look like a firestorm came through, cutting down most everything standing. From the point of view of the seed, wherever there is soil, there is opportunity.

Life has more tricks up her sleeve than any of us will ever know in our lifetime—serotiny being one of them. What other seeds are in the soil, waiting to sprout—be they mustard seeds of faith or fireweed of youth or even ancient seeds from a previous interglacial period?

Knowing this, even hope seems too small a ground to stand on. I now have trust. Hope allows us to act with expectancy. Trust allows us to relax into what is, into the resilience of life itself. Hope is our relationship with the future. Trust is our relationship with the eternal present. Hope lets us try. Trust gives us assurance that we are not inventing but rather cooperating with forces more powerful than our little human wills.

It is in this spirit of trust that I invite you to read on. To ask, "How can I, where I live, engage in this work of food system restoration?" You'll be cooperating with a movement that's growing, well, like weeds. Young people in droves want to farm now. In fact, most of the young people I now know consider my generation and me the fireweed and lodgepole pines. They are about to grow a new forest.

Mapping a Food System

Here's an overview of the work of restoring regional food systems. As the Island County food system report mentioned earlier reveals, there is more to a system than farms and farmers and eaters.

These are the typical food system elements—whether industrial or complementary:

- Farm suppliers that provide seed, compost, starts, equipment, and more to gardeners and farmers

- Farmers, large and small, growing for subscription customers, for farmers' markets, for chefs and stores
- Enterprises that process and package produce and meats
- Slaughterhouses and butchers where local grass-fed animals become the shrink-wrapped, frozen, and canned foods we can buy retail (or process a quarter of an animal for our freezer)
- Markets, from farm stands to farmers' markets to grocery stores
- Distributors, from personalized delivery services to warehouses and food hubs

These elements are usually put in a line—the food value chain—starting not with seeds but with harvest and ending not with compost but at the checkout counter. Life's cycles don't count. Only the business cycles. Relational eaters know that the value chain is just a delivery system, not a food system. We need to put nature back in as the context and culture back in as the major driver.

The Butcher, the Baker, the Candlestick Maker

Culture is in a way the "customer" of this food system. It's our human preferences, social customs, religious taboos, and economic structures. It is eaters, but it is also how people in their social and professional roles influence the system. Once you see the variety of actors who affect our food choices, you see how much power we each have in shaping our food future.

Here's my list of system transformers:

• The eaters—that would be all of us—who grow, cook, share, dine, educate, promote, lobby, fund, donate, and are the ultimate customers for what this amazing system produces.

• The markets, large and small, that stock local food and farmers' markets and farm stands and CSAs that bring us produce cut and washed at dawn.

• The market makers that brand and promote. The industrial system is great at this piece of the food puzzle! People internalize product jingles and develop brand loyalty.

• The nonprofits that support local and organic and homegrown and artisan values and protect farmland and support young people learning to farm. They research legislation, develop business incubators, and engage in land preservation.

• The educators, who teach, write, and speak about food, gardening, and food systems. Michael Pollan seems to be the current educator-in-chief for local food, but there are literally countless K-16 courses about food, systems, politics, good practices, and more. *Mother Earth News* is the grandmother journal, but just the other day I saw a new magazine at the grocery checkout called *Urban Farmer*.

• The activists who challenge the system, muckrake, expose, and advocate for change. This advocacy space is full and getting larger as groups and individuals press against the "get big or get out" agricultural orthodoxy. Every issue is on the table: safety, sovereignty, transparency, justice, conservation, ownership, subsidies, education, security, sufficiency. Every issue has dozens of champions, heroes, bulldogs, and educators. Progress is slow but the pressure is implacable.

• The financiers, large and small: the credit unions, banks, donors, investors, and lenders who help small enterprises get off the ground and grow.

• The chefs who serve their customers local food and teach people to use local ingredients through restaurants as well as culinary schools, community colleges, adult education classes, online videos, and gourmet magazines.

• The institutions that feed their students, patients, and residents in schools, hospitals, and cafeterias—and are eager to serve fresh, natural, wholesome foods. They are making markets for local products at a rapid pace.

• The event producers that celebrate and uphold local food, county fairs, and community potlucks.

• The food banks that grow, glean, buy, and receive donations of fresh food.

An Agenda for We the Eaters

Understanding the food system and understanding who the transformers are, I could come back to those resolves I made to bless the hands that feed me here on Whidbey. In chapter 6 I enumerated them. Now I reviewed them:

1. Get farmland into the hands of young and new dedicated farmers . . . or at least get them reliable, affordable, and long-term secure access to farmland that they can invest themselves in and reap the rewards from for years to come.

2. Do something about the cost difference between local food and industrial food. Buy local—not only farm produce but milk and meat, jams and jellies, canned dilly beans, and such.

3. Yes, regulate the industrial system. Protect supermarket shoppers who want to think only about what's for dinner, not where it came from . . . but make "scale-appropriate" regulations for the little local guys.

4. Inform myself—and others. Get up off my consumerism laurels and learn enough to really help.

5. Do that 50 percent within fifty miles in February. Rise at least to the challenge of a local winter diet.

I am pleased to see how much progress I've made. Number five is done and the result is that I am now a year-round local eater when possible. Item four is in your hands. This book arises from that resolve, as well as whatever I write or speak about from this day forward.

Now for the tough stuff. Items one to three.

There are two policy directions in the United States that I believe are crucial to seed and cultivate the flourishing regional food systems of the future. They aren't a full agenda, just two levers we can pull to change the flow of events and the course of history:

1. **Scale-appropriate regulations,** which would liberate neighbor-to-neighbor trade from the regulations and fees imposed to protect the national food supply. People who raise animals for their milk and eggs and people who raise, slaughter, and butcher animals for home consumption and sell livestock would be able to sell to people they know. This is community-based food security, with performance-based measures (is the food healthy?) rather than production-based regulations (is the milking parlor painted correctly?). People growing food for their neighbors need to be seen as Good Samaritans, not as outlaws.

There is already a "cottage laws" movement to legalize selling "non--potentially-hazardous foods"—like baked goods, jams, candies, fruit pies, herb blends, dried fruits, granola, etc.—made in home kitchens. Such laws exist, to one degree or another, in thirty-one states. They liberate entry-level food entrepreneurs to market-test their OMG-is-that-delicious! recipes—some just at farmers' markets and neighbor to neighbor, some in retail outlets if all labeling and licensing requirements are met. It reduces red tape and excessive fees while still assuring a product as safe as commercial-kitchen-made.

What about milk? Aah, now you have a food fight, because arguments rage about the safety of raw milk. It's useful to compare countries rather than states in the United States, because that reveals different culinary sensibilities and rights around the world. The European Union, for example, deems all raw milk products safe for human consumption. The same goes for Asia, Africa, England, Wales and Northern Ireland, and New Zealand. In France it goes further: raw milk is de rigueur for cheese.

And meat? According to the Washington State University Extension, the USDA exempts from federal oversight farmers who butcher for resale up to one thousand birds (chickens and turkeys) a year, whether on the farm or at what are called "custom cut" slaughterhouses.[6] How this exemption is interpreted varies from state to state, but where I live the state is lenient, meaning the home-butchered chickens I bought were legal. But the custom cuts of beef from Long's had to be butchered in a USDA-approved facility—on the mainland—to be legal.

Progress is slow in liberating niche-market meats—pasture-raised, organic, local beef, lamb, goat, and pig—from Draconian regulations designed for large slaughterhouses that process thousands of animals daily. Only the four largest meat processors—which butcher more than 80 percent of our meat—can afford the costs of licensing, and of constructing and managing facilities, and of paying USDA inspectors, and of testing each animal to the letter of the law. The little guys can't. Fortunately, we have farmers like the Longs and 3 Sisters who jump through the hoops, but it seems that the kind of laws that apply to chickens can eventually apply to other meats, making neighbor-to-neighbor sale legal—and bringing down the cost.

Independent farmers and ranchers by and large dislike regulations. They believe they know more about their business, and do it to a higher standard, than the regulators do. They resent the costs, which make it harder to compete in the marketplace. There's a natural libertarian streak here—and I have it too. That's why I'm keeping an eye out for how to free neighbor-to-neighbor trade from the cloak of illegality while still upholding the need for uniform, enforced standards when we purchase from industrial producers. Having lived here a long time, I can avail myself of those rivers of sustenance that flow through the community, but eventually such relational trade should be available to anyone willing to hold their neighbors harmless, and see the food more like loaves and fishes and less like plastic-wrapped packages stamped with bar codes.

2. In addition to liberating local trade, **we need to liberate the thousands of young people who want to farm** from the systemic shackles that render them instantly impoverished and often doomed if they choose farming over, say, joining the ranks of corporate employees. So many factors—from corporate money to our habituation to cheap food—devalue small-scale farming and thus farmers. Earlier I cited a statistic that should frighten any eater: less than 2 percent of Americans now farm, and their average age is nearly sixty. Who will farm your food in ten years—especially if you favor

sustainably produced fare? Who will produce the food in your four-hundred-mile circle from home?

My proposal mirrors two massive post–World War II programs designed to get the Western world on its feet and humming again: the Marshall Plan in Europe and the GI Bill in the United States. In Europe, the task was to rebuild infrastructure—and morale—after the devastation and decimation of war. In the United States, the task was to employ returning GIs, giving them a leg up so they could root their military victory in the healthy soil of a shared prosperity.

Among the benefits of the GI Bill were low-cost mortgages, loans to start a business or farm, financial support to attend high school, college, or vocational education, plus unemployment compensation for a year.

Translate that to young farmers and you get low-cost mortgages to buy farms, loans for start-up costs for a market garden or CSA, financial support for vocational training in sustainable farming, plus a year of living expenses posttraining to tide them over until the farm is closer to operating in the black. In fact, returning vets are also interested in farming, so this would literally be a GI Bill all over again.

The effect would be like a Marshall Plan for young farmers: correct the devastation our policies have had on community-scale farms and the livelihoods of farmers—decimating the growing profession—and build the capacity of our regional food systems to nourish us at the 50 percent level at least. That's twelve hundred calories a day. That's survival.

Here's the wish list I put together. Some of them are already under way, and perhaps by publication will be even more robust. Some of them seem nigh on to impossible, but it's a wish list, not (yet) a to-do list.

- Secure tenure on land young farmers can farm—be it leasing or buying or gifting
- Apprenticeships with experienced farmers

- Scholarships for college and training programs
- Debt forgiveness from undergraduate student loans for people entering farming as a profession
- Low-interest loans and grants for seeds and equipment to get started
- Some clever strategies to help their hand-raised food compete in the mechanically-raised food marketplace
- Health insurance
- Crop insurance, just like the big guys
- To know—through honors and awards—that we value their efforts
- All of us working toward regulations that support family and mid-size farms

The "how" of this list showed up when I met Severine von Tscharner Fleming. She is a farmer in upstate New York and the sassy, confident, funny, and informed cofounder of the Greenhorns, a network of young farmers who provide mutual support while developing kick-ass policies that they take to Washington. She was on a panel at a conference. She seemed distracted. Her mat of curly light brown hair looked a bit like a wren's nest. When she spoke, though, she was at once rat-a-tat ruthless in her political analysis and endearing in her offhand humor. Even the Greenhorns' literature feels young-farmer funky: line drawings (and not that good) and not an ounce of slick. I'd found my primo informant on my quest to support my young island farmers—and attract more.

The Greenhorns intend to shift the systemic conditions that make farming tough—including dating! How are you going to meet someone who wants to live down on the farm between milking, tilling, weeding, doing the books, and on and on. The Greenhorns have weed dating—working while flirting. They surveyed young farmers and found out what irked, bugged, and stumped them. They were the same needs I'd seen in the lives of my farmers: access to capital and credit, access to affordable land, education and training, business expertise, and health-care coverage.

Not only that, the Greenhorns have a policy agenda that is no wimpy wish list. Severine rattled off how international trade and anemic national support for sustainable food and farming and overproduction of commodity crops all link. Awareness, she said, is not enough—though it's a starting point. Individual action is necessary—but not sufficient. We need an analysis of these systemic relationships and we need concerted action toward policies that integrate agriculture with the earth's living systems.

Sounds like relational agriculture to me. And agriculture in context.

When I asked her how I and people like me—not young, not farmers—can help, she at first gave the standard line about farmers' markets and CSAs, but when I pressed and she got that I was determined, she rattled off what young farmers need from boomer eaters. Here's the list—my list and, if you choose, your list:

- Providing funding in the form of loans, gifts, and investments
- Helping out with the ancillary tasks of farming, such as marketing, Web site, and business planning
- Activating our established networks of influence to help open doors they can't
- Passing on the institutional knowledge on how to navigate the system learned during our own long careers
- Listening, coaching, celebrating, admiring, and other forms of social support
- Offering land with long tenure or generous terms
- Helping to campaign and lobby and sticking with the long slog of change
- Using our own capital, business skills, and clout to build the intermediate infrastructure for distribution and processing
- Acting in a spirit of collaboration rather than "helping"—be in it together

Hearing this was actually energizing. She confirmed my gut sense. The Greenhorns' agenda, if it was adopted whole hog, so to speak, would turn the tide on Whidbey and probably on every region of the country. I now had a road map for contribution that could last me a lifetime and leave a legacy for the new eaters currently growing up.

It can be your game too. We are all eaters. We've all bent our elbows millions of times to put tons of food into our mouths. Eating unites us as a species among species on a living earth. Relational eating can unite us in making safe, affordable, abundant, healthy, and fair food in a way we care with and for one another—and the future.

This now, for me, is the great adventure: revitalizing our regional food systems, thriving together. It is, as one of my spiritual teachers put it years ago, a game worth playing. It has all the elements: risk, challenge, uncertainty, and celebration of the daily wins with no idea what's coming next.

Your Food Map

In the beginning of the book I introduced the food map. You traveled with me as I mapped mine. Now it's your turn to stand in the middle of your food world and discover the hands and lands that feed you.

Recall that insight that food isn't "out there," it's all around us. Our food sources ripple out in every direction from where we stand—from our yards to our communities to our regions to our nations to our world.

Let's investigate your relationship with each widening circle of your food map, and with the hands and lands that feed *you*.

The center of your food map is within you in your heart—your inner relationship with food. That includes your history, culture, assumptions, beliefs, preferences, and motivations to change. If transformation is going to happen, it starts here.

The first ring is your household food system. *This is what's on your shelves and in your fridge, the tools you have, and the way you cook and shop*. It also includes you the farmer—the sprouts on the windowsill, the tomatoes on your patio, or the garden plot in your yard. It's easy to make changes here—cook more, grow more, shop wiser.

Around your intimate one-to-one relationship with growing and gathering food is your community food system—the fields and forests, markets, stores, and farm stands. It includes your farmers, ranchers, butchers, processors, packagers, and merchants within an hour of home. These are the hands and lands you can touch, feel, wander, and smell.

There are so many choices we can make to patronize, promote, and produce for our food neighborhood. You may still buy just three beets a week at the farmers' market, but you now understand how it all fits together.

Your regional food system is the next ring out. I call it USDA local—four hundred miles, give or take a few hundred. How much of what you can't get in your neighborhood can you get in your region? This can be a treasure hunt. Can you get all the fruit you want? Salt, sweetener, spices, vinegars, and even oil? Can you get all your meat? All your vegetables? Even your flours and beans and grains?

Transition Colorado—fired up by a visionary spark plug, Michael Brownlee—is systematically moving toward sourcing 25 percent of Boulder County's food locally. Their Local Food Shift Campaign' is "working to help shift our food and farming system—our foodshed—towards significantly increased production and consumption of locally-grown, locally-produced, and locally-sourced foods." They commissioned Michael Shuman, Mr. Economic Relocalization himself, and found "that this 25% shift could create 1,899 new jobs, providing work for more than one in seven unemployed residents. It could increase annual wages in the county by $81 million, gross county product by $138 million, and state and local business taxes by $12 million." They are taking a multiprong approach to this shift, increasing both production capacity and consumer demand as well as rebuilding the local food shed infrastructure. This gives food system activists both courage and a road map for success. And we need it.

If you think in terms of bioregions or food sheds—defining your food circle by geography and ecology rather than miles—this ring may extend a thousand miles, as my Cascadia region does, from Northern California to British Columbia. It actually makes more sense to measure nature by nature, not by a human invention like miles—but as eaters whose food comes in via roads and rails, "food miles" feeds our civilized imaginations. To talk in bioregion or food shed is like learning a new language or entering a different culture.

Beyond your regional food system are your state and national systems and the agencies and political landscape that govern big policies like subsidies, conservation, food safety, trade, favored agricultural practices, grants, and crops. These profoundly influence how difficult it is and will be to build the health, vitality, and fertility of our regional systems. Before my 10-mile diet, did I know anything about the U.S. Farm Bill, the USDA, the FDA, and other agencies and regulators affecting what shows up on my neatly ordered grocery store shelves? Nope. Did I know the link between agriculture and climate destabilization, peak oil, resource depletion, and erosion? Barely. It was of interest, but not of consequence—and very easy to ignore.

GROWING COMMUNITIES IN THE UK

Searching for answers to "Can we feed the world? Can the world feed itself? Does local matter?" I came upon a project in the UK that literally maps on this map I offer you. Growing Communities in Hackney has done the down-and-dirty work of creating a model of local to regional food systems that can indeed nourish people, lands, communities, and hearts. If you want to work on re-regionalizing your food system, theirs is a solid set of principles and actions.

Growing Communities is a social enterprise committed to providing a safe, abundant, affordable alternative to the industrial food system for the people of Hackney, East London, through community-led trade. A small group there asked the question I had asked: "Can our island—theirs being the UK—feed ourselves?"

They function like a food hub, collectively using the buying power of their community to purchase fresh produce from many area farms, as well as growing some of their own on city plots. Members pick up their "Veg Box" weekly, and also shop at a farmers' market. The enterprise is run democratically—everyone, from farmers to employees, gets paid a fair wage—and they are in the black.

As they grow and prosper they are refining a set of interconnected principles that are, they will readily admit, a work in progress and often involve trade-offs. These are the properties of a sustainable and resilient food system (words in parentheses are mine):

- Involve food farmed and produced "ecologically" (without chemicals, promoting natural fertility)
- Involve mainly plant-based food (which is far more likely to provide food security for the community)
- Involve fresh/minimally processed food (reducing the energy costs of processing and maximizing nutrition)
- Involve trade between appropriately scaled operations (small plots for salad, larger plots for vegetables—scaling sideways between equal players)
- Increase the consumption of food sourced as locally, seasonally and directly as practicable (leaning into a complementary food system)
- Use resources in an environmentally friendly and low carbon way (doing the least damage to the living systems)
- Trade fairly (allowing everyone involved to have a fair shake and a living wage)
- Be transparent and promote trust throughout the food chain (revealing sources and practices)
- Promote knowledge (empowering customers to become informed and engaged)
- Foster community (members meet their neighbors when they collect their Veg Boxes at a common pickup point—relational eating!)
- Strive to be economically viable and independent (standing on its own feet as an enterprise)
- Enshrine the principles in everything it does (acting with integrity at every step of the value chain)[8]

These principles are expressed in a series of rings around one's home, much like the one I suggest with the eater in the middle and concentric circles of household, neighborhood, community, region, and beyond. Their vision is food resilience for urban areas.

They call the center zone Zero, which is your household. They imagine you can provide 2.5 percent of your food through your own garden.

Zone 1 is urban traded—salads, leafy greens, fruit—providing another 5 percent.

Zone 2 is peri-urban (the suburbs) land, where field-scale produce, staples, and chickens might grow. They presume you can source 17.5 percent from there.

Zone 3 is what they call the rural hinterland, a one-hundred-mile circle where another 35 percent of food is grown. There they presume livestock for eggs, milk, cheese, and meat are grown as well as substantial field crops. As you can see, they calculate, as do I, that it's feasible to provide 50 percent within one hundred miles. Farther afield—for them the rest of the UK and out to the rest of Europe—you have livestock, orchards, and the plentiful foods that grow well in other regions. From the rest of the world you get your exotics.

And beyond your nation is the rest of the world, where much of our food grows because economics and transportation make it so easy to use the land and labor of other regions to stock our shelves. Here you as an eater may have little direct influence, but you can vote with your dollars, and you can inform yourself about global food politics. Ask: Is it fair? Are people faring well? Why or why not? What are the stories of despair—and of hope? Once you care about relational eating, you pretty much care about everything and everyone.

Finally, there is the natural world that hums with life and from which all food comes. It has no distance because it is everywhere! We call it "the environment" and it begins probably in our guts with intestinal bacteria and extends into the upper atmosphere, through forests and rivers, jungles and oceans, ponds and savannas. Billions upon billions of eaters live here, all kin. Protecting "nature" isn't just a sweet afterthought, a virtue. Assuring enough for all species actually assures enough for humans. To paraphrase the famous Martin Niemuller quote about the Church's inaction as the Nazis vilified and arrested first the Communists, then the unionists, then the Jews, and so Christians had "no one left to speak for them" when they were taken, we need to protect the whole system else our food systems fail us with no backups from the vast wealth of species. Climate becomes a food issue. The rights of nature is a food issue. Relational eating is a lens that brings into focus how our lives are woven into the whole web of life.

You don't need to think about this every day before breakfast. But you might!

For every ring of your food system map—personal, community, region, and beyond—there are practices to engage in, projects to do, policies to advocate for. Because it is a system, not just a laundry list of good ideas or new right ways to do things, you know that your small acts are part of something intimate, yet—through networking—vast. You can eat a local rutabaga, you can start a food policy council, you can click a link to sign a petition, you can volunteer at the food bank, you can join a CSA, you can move your money to a credit union that lends to local businesses, you can order the local burger on the menu, you can plant a seed, you can invite a friend to dinner. Food is everywhere! Food is literally in your face many times a day. You can put yourself "in" food again. Be part of what is growing.

This food map, from inner to global, is the context for all the following action steps.

Now It's Your Turn: Discovering the Hands That Feed You

Get to Know Your Food Shed Better by Asking These Questions:

- What are the boundaries of my version of "local"? A USDA four-hundred-mile circle might not be quite right. You might choose a bioregion, a state, a watershed, an island.

- Is "here" where I want to be in ten years? Am I willing to inhabit "here" as a relational eater? If not, then where?
- What grows well in my region, in nature, in farms, and in backyard gardens?
- How many of the foods I commonly eat are available from my region? Who supplies each one of them?
- How far do I need to go for the rest of my common foods? By what criteria will I choose each of these?
- Who are my farmers? Find a dozen growers, large and small, in your region and acquaint yourself with them by reading or shopping or visiting.

Once You've Discovered the Answers, Set Yourself Some Tasks:

- Commit to what percent of your food you will source from your region (1 percent is okay—you can always go to 2 percent next year).
- Make field trips—literally! Visit nearby farms.
- Commit to one farmer. Buy her food as a matter of relationship. Learn about his life sufficiently to understand the joys and challenges of farming and how you might help—beyond buying—to have his family flourish. Hear about her challenges. If you "adopt" a regional farmer in this intimate way, you will find yourself in widening circles of community care.
- Commit to one food that grows well in your region and learn about it. Where does it like to grow? What family is it in? How many ways can you cook it? What are its beneficial properties—both nutritionally and medicinally? How did the native peoples prepare it?

From these queries and commitments you will become ever more intimate with the hands and lands that feed you.

No final recipe. Instead Jess Dowdell offered to share a seasonal menu she created for the Whidbey Island Farm Tour. I wanted you to see how a many-course local menu, prepared with love and skill by a relational chef, can be as elegant and flavorful as that of any five-star restaurant in the centers of haute cuisine.

September 14, 2012

WHIDBEY ISLAND FARM TOUR DINNER

CHEF JESS DOWDELL, ROAMING RADISH

FIRST COURSE

Paired with Spoiled Dog Pinot Gris

Pickled beet and carrot bruschetta, Whidbey Island herbed goat chèvre, and lavender crostini

[Willowood Farm, Quail's Run Farm, Little Brown Farm, Lavender Wind Farm]

SECOND COURSE

Paired with Spoiled Dog Estate Rose of Pinot Noir

Fennel, apple, and arugula salad dressed with parsley pesto

Organic red quinoa

[Quail's Run Farm, Willowood Farm]

THIRD COURSE

Paired with Spoiled Dog Pinot Noir

Summer quinoa tabbouleh with cucumbers, tomato, mint, and shallots

[Quail's Run Farm]

Roasted lamb shoulder

[Glendale Shepherd]

Polenta croutons

[Quail's Run Farm]

Fire-roasted peppers, onions, and tomatoes

[Quail's Run Farm, Willowood Farm]

Island Brebis raw sheep cheese

[Glendale Shepherd]

FOURTH COURSE

Paired with Spoiled Dog Deception Red

Chocolate decadence with blueberry reduction, made with loganberry liqueur

Organic Sunspire chocolate

[Huntersmoon Blueberries, Whidbey Island Distillery]

Continued Blessing

It's over two years since I was released from my 10-mile diet and liberated into toast, nuts, avocados, and more. Or thought I'd been set free, as if freedom were the willful ability to do as you please.

These intervening years of researching and writing, listening and inquiring, eating emmer and potatoes, kale and barley, chicken and beef, milk and eggs, summer greens and winter roots—all from Whidbey—have heaped on me those other freedoms that come from rooting, from being nourished without effort because you belong. When you belong you are not confined, but rather confirmed by others as part of their lives. You have a home—and a home team.

Surprising Side Benefit of the 10-Mile Diet

The benefits of this belonging are far more than a secure supper or even a circle of friends. For me, the diet has led to solving a seemingly different set of problems—those that come from aging in a transient culture.

In these two years since that Maxwelton Beach Fourth of July potluck, I've rounded the bend from age sixty-four to sixty-seven . . . going on seventy, going on that late fall time in life when—like leaves falling from trees—things fall away from us: jowls sink off the chin line, and you lose height, teeth, and even ambition. Mind you, I don't—yet—act my age, but I have had to consider what I need to do now to be sure the near-carcass I'll be living in twenty years from now (should I get there) will be comfortable and cared for.

The dancer Anna Halprin says, "Old age is enlightenment at

gunpoint." Perhaps it's the ultimate extreme sport. I don't intend to do it warehoused in a "facility" paid for by "long-term-care insurance." If money is our safety net, in this economy that's no safety at all. I used to say "I want to die with a dime in my pocket, but not a day later."

How, though, does one manage that? How much of my stored resource called money do I need to conserve now to conserve my stored resource called a body for an unknown number of years? Clever as I am, I had not been able to solve this puzzle—until the 10-mile diet. As I enact "belonging" and "community" day by day, week by week, I can be confident that on those days in the future when I need help, someone here will probably drive me to the doctor or bring by a meal. Wendell Berry talks of this freedom of community. The people and community in his novels, woven and polished by long association, have the feel of a bygone era: nostalgic, fragile, precious. What if relational eating—the local food movement—is a precursor of a new era of belonging, when once again homeland security will mean neighbors, not an increasing dependency on a militaristic state? What if turning our attention to "here-ing" through bringing our eating closer to home is not just a good way to eat but also a wise way to age? Perhaps a culture of permanence provides more true freedom than a culture of transience.

Am I becoming a fuddy-duddy? I don't think so. I think I am simply getting the hang of living. God, it takes so long!

Blessing Itself

Like the 10-mile-diet caper itself, I picked the title *Blessing the Hands That Feed Us* on a whim. I thought it was just a clever play on "biting the hands that feed you"—a phrase that means ingratitude toward your benefactors.

As I wrote, however, I realized how profound the act of blessing is, how far it goes. Now the "hands that feed me" include the organisms in the soil, the bees that spread pollen, the birds that spread seeds, and the forests where the mycelium of chanterelles grows in darkness until conditions are right for the mushrooms to appear.

The "hands" now also means the miraculous dynamism of nature itself—how the sun warms the surface, driving cycles of wind and rain while bestowing the very energy green plants need to make chlorophyll. The hands are not just the farmer's hands, but the truck driver's and the grocer's and the researchers and the teachers who pass on knowledge to young people so the whole growing cycles can continue.

To bless doesn't just mean "think good thoughts" or "be nice." To bless is far more radical. It is to actually give life, to have one's cup run over into the lives of others. To have one's parents' blessings is to have each of them send you off into life saying "I see you. I know you are good. I believe in you. I trust you. I am proud of you. May you be fruitful and multiply, whatever that means to you." To bless is to speak from and for and to the divine, as a priest blesses a marriage or christens a baby. To bless is to respect the integrity and mystery of the life of another.

And this holiness is what I sense through buying, cooking, and eating real food grown by real people in real places. My farmers.

Where Are My Farmers and Friends Now?

Last season Tricia and Kent launched a Friday Farmers' Market in downtown Langley, a festive end-of-the-week opportunity to stroll among booths where Eric Conn and Vicky Brown and Tricia and Molly and John Peterson pile up their week's produce. Sadly for me, though, they just sold their property to a young couple eager to make a sustainable farming life here. I had, of course, hoped they would be a permanent fixture in my eating life, but life going on means change. Maybe these new people will become as dear to me as Tricia and Kent. Life going on also means that new folks will arrive to fill your heart. And happily for me, life going on for Tricia and Kent was buying a fixer-upper half a mile from me as the crow flies.

Pam will still be able to farm her half of Tricia and Kent's production garden; that was part of the deal. She continues to be an amazing grower and saleswoman and now has a winter crop too: knitted caps and scarves.

Britt and Eric now have a beautiful baby boy whom I adore as if he were my own. Their farm as well as family is expanding, a new plot of veggies planted where we'd planted our tables two years ago at the wedding.

Georgie Smith is flourishing and I'm proud to have a small hand in that. In another search for a solution to a relocalization issue—local finance—I'd come across a model for local lending from Port Townsend, across the water from Whidbey. The Local Investing Opportunity Network formed several years ago for that very purpose. They researched the strict SEC laws, passed to protect investors from buying swampland in Florida, and came up with a model for connecting potential businesses with potential investors without being considered investment advisers or an investment club. I called it back then "speed dating for lending"—just a way to meet and mate (financially, that is). I heard that Georgie needed money to build a greenhouse, and we sat down for coffee in Coupeville so I could convince her that I was on the up-and-up about investing in her farm. We struck a deal: several thousand dollars for the greenhouse, paid back over three years, with the interest paid in vegetables rather than money. In weeks the greenhouse was up. I've enjoyed a year of Rockwell beans and specialty garlic, and the loan is almost repaid.

Lynn Willeford, my superb local editor-cum-metaphor-pruner, got wind of that LION model at the same time I did, and in her superb low-key but effective community-organizing way she, her husband, Blake, and another couple got our Whidbey Island Local Lending (W.I.L.L.) going.

Speaking of lending, Jess Dowdell, formerly of the Ca'buni café at Mukilteo Coffee Roasters, has opened the Roaming Radish, a deli and catering establishment plus cooking school, featuring her same stable of local growers and foods. She organized the chefs on the island to provide the recipes at the end of each chapter. I only love her more—for her spunk and drive and high standards for the ingredients she uses.

Vicky Brown, the goat cheese maven, sought a different kind of funding for a cheese cave where she can age cheese for a harder, sharper product. She used Kickstarter, an online tool for raising money for projects, which resulted in 270 backers, $22,678 funded— well over goal. In an interview on the Marcella the Cheesemonger site she says: "With 5 days left (53 days from the start of the project) we weren't even 60% to our goal. The interesting thing about Kickstarter is you only fund your project if you hit your goal. It wasn't looking good. Then there was . . . neighbors and friends forwarding links like crazy through social media. Suddenly we hit our goal with 26 hours to spare! . . . Before the last week, I had already started to recognize the true value of our campaign. Although the funding was awesome and spectacular, that wasn't the largest benefit. The real benefit was feeling the community (from neighbors to cheese lovers in Denmark) support in a concrete and tangible way."

Are Vicky and I bosom buddies? Given that we are both of "traditional build," as Alexander McCall Smith labeled his heroine in the No. 1 Ladies' Detective Agency series, we could be such buddies, but we are mostly cheerfully supportive of each other, echoing "Hi Vicki/y" several times each time we see each other.

Quiet, dedicated innovator Maryon Attwood has moved on from Greenbank Farm but not from her passion for integrating the food system on Whidbey. She convened a group to discuss buying a grain mill for Whidbey to support existing grain growers and hopefully attract others to growing grains. The idea has not yet ripened, but the seed is sown. Not one to be idle, Maryon is now working with her partner, Robbie Lobell, in another part of the food system: they make clay ovenware. The company is called Cooked on Clay, and if we imagine Whidbey Island being more self-sufficient it's good to know we can make our own pots and pans.

Speaking of Greenbank Farm and the New Farmer Training

Program, two graduates—Annie Jesperson and Nathaniel Talbot—graduated but stayed put. She is a social worker by training, he's a musician, but their desire and destiny is to farm together. They established a winter vegetable CSA, which inspired Cary Peterson of the Good Cheer Food Bank Garden to create a program, Fresh Food for the Table, so that people in need can have veggies all winter. A yearly fund-raiser brought in enough money to pay them for a season.

Then Annie and Nathaniel sent a message over the local tom-toms (a unique daily list of South Whidbey opportunities for work, play, and swapping) that they wanted to rent or lease or simply have access to a farm. Meanwhile, Molly and John Peterson's daughter, Anna, decided to go to Sebhory in Guinea and now Annie and Nathaniel are farming part of Molly and John's land and cathedral-sized greenhouses.

The teacher who enlightened me about soil fertility is biodynamic farmer Chris Korrow, who, with his wife, Christy, have moved in down the hill from me and become a real anchor for my sense of home and community. They came from Kentucky a year ago, sad to leave their ninety-acre farm but glad to be among people who share their values. Chris is an author, filmmaker, and philosopher as well as a farmer, and we often talk through the fence between the community garden where I have a plot and his fields where he raises winter vegetables. He has "that something" that makes the green world want to grow. I joke about his crisp plate-sized spinach leaves, saying that if they were an animal they would bite me. Same with the squash, green beans, broccoli. I feel fortunate that a few minutes away I can have fresh-picked nutritious vegetables every day thanks to his efforts and skill.

The undercover milkers—goat and cow—are still unfortunately undercover. A bill is ambling through the Washington state legislature. Senator Kevin Ranker is sponsoring Senate Bill 5648, which adds a section to the law regulating direct sales of milk, which stipulates that if the milk is not advertised for sale and produced on a small-scale farm where there are no more than two producing dairy cows, nine producing sheep, or nine producing goats, it can be sold directly to customers.

That about covers all my hyperlocal suppliers and is a model for what I mean by "scale-appropriate regulation."

And here I am, raising my eyes off the screen and the page to begin the long journey of accompanying this toddler book out into the world. I joked when I got the contract that it was a "late-in-life pregnancy." I hadn't expected to birth anything bigger than a local project (see above about the falling away of ambition), but I feel blessed to have this opportunity to do good world work again.

In fact, deepening into understanding all the dimensions of relational eating will take years. It's a long journey from being disconnected from our sources of nourishment to experiencing ourselves as fully part of nature. Nature isn't "out there"—someplace to go on a weekend. As food, nature is coursing through us. Our guts and the soils are intertwined, both alive with microorganisms doing the work of transforming organic matter into strong plants, trees, and bodies.

Likewise, it will take decades to deepen into understanding how I, a relational eater, can influence the future of food for this earth—or at least for my geographic and cultural food region. As I begin to develop knowledge of the food movements, I am heartened to see how my personal tale fits. At a 2013 conference on organic standards, I left the dinner table to get a dessert (a definitely not local chocolate confection). When I came back, I had a new tablemate, Laura Ridenour. We chatted and I discovered that she, like me, is interested in food systems and social change. Laura is a twenty-year food system activist, and she's become my educator in chief, informing me how local relational eating is part of the broad engagement in "civic agriculture"—place-based eating—and how "food democracy"—empowers individuals and communities toward a place-based, participatory food system. I've discovered that there are many lenses for food activism—fair, safe, local, organic, healthy, real, nontoxic—but not all the lenses are necessarily aligned and focused on a shared goal. There's a real ferment at the moment of strategies and ideas. They are old—echoing the Jeffersonian agrarian and populist appeals—and they are a new uprising *against* corporate-controlled agriculture and *for* restoring our connections with the hands and lands that feed us.

The more I learn, the happier I am that I get to be part of this for the rest of my life. It is my privilege to know a little more and care a lot more and so be willing to learn and act on behalf of the fertility of the soils, the vitality of the wild, and the health of our food systems.

How odd and grand to have followed a thin thread of interest only to find myself woven into the web of life.

Acknowledgments

I'll be brief in offering my gratitudes because if I go beyond those materially involved in this book I'll have to thank multitudes of people going back many years. First, I want to say thank you to Tricia Beckner, my "feeder" for the 10-mile diet. Little did you know, Tricia, that your casual idea would take root in me and grow this book and change my life. We never know what chance encounter will change our lives, do we? Beth Vesel, my agent, is another agent of change. She sought out Joe Dominguez and me nearly twenty-five years ago after reading a magazine article about us. Beth sold us on writing *Your Money or Your Life,* then sold the proposal to Viking. Ever since she has believed in me as a writer and thinker with more to say. Kathryn Court, my editor at Viking Penguin, has been a staunch supporter and has gently given me clues as to what works and what doesn't.

Now I feel like I'm accepting an Oscar because I'm going to gush that I could not have developed the narrative of this book without Lynn Willeford, my local editor. While we share values we have polar opposite personalities—she cuts to the chase, I never met a metaphor I couldn't jam into a sentence somewhere. In fact, she doesn't much like me gushing over her. Nonetheless, it's true that I often needed her skillful surgery; she gave me unvarnished feedback that improved this book immensely. My muse and champion was—and still is— Deborah Nedelman, my writing partner. We've kept a weekly writing date since the spring of 2010. We write in silence for several hours, read aloud, offer almost homeopathic feedback that pulls the essence of the piece out. The routine has kept us both going. It turned out that both her adult children are interested in sustainable food systems and in fact her daughter Eden met with me weekly via Skype when I first got the contract to help me babble into clarity about what I really wanted to say through my story. Thank you, Eden.

Here's where other people thank their partners for patience, kindness, forbearance, editing, and taking care of the kids and dinner. I, however, live alone with my cat, and she's offered none of that kind of support. I will say that many wonderful friends and neighbors here on Whidbey heard me out when I was piecing things together, and the local farmers and chefs in this book graciously responded to my questions and reviewed my stories. I could also single out Comedy Island, my improv troupe, that cheered me on and got me to fall on the floor laughing week in and week out. And Mel Watson's weekly meditation class reminded me that I am not a writer, really, but a soul traversing lifetimes.

We call people like these godsends and I think that the divine has been sending me such guides, helpers, goads, and cheerleaders my whole life. I am profoundly grateful for the ones who showed up to help with this book and feel a shiver of anticipation as I think that more godsends are coming to send me on more holy adventures.

Notes

Introduction

1. J. C. Rickman, D. M. Barrett, and C. M. Bruhn, "Nutritional Comparison of Fresh, Frozen and Canned Fruits and Vegetables, Part I, Vitamins C and B and Phenolic Compounds," *Journal of the Science of Food and Agriculture* 87 (2007): 930–44.

Chapter One: Localize Me?

1. "Diet (nutrition)," *Wikipedia,* last modified December 2, 2012, http://en.wikipedia.org/wiki/Diet_%28nutrition%29.

Chapter Three: Yes! But How?

1. Greg Lange, "Native Americans force settlers to leave Whidbey Island in August 1848," HistoryLink.org Essay 5246, last modified February 19, 2003, http://www.historylink.org/index.cfm?DisplayPage-output.cfm&file_id=5246.

2 Andrew L. Stoll, *The Omega-3 Connection: The Groundbreaking Anti-depression Diet and Brain Program* (New York: Simon & Schuster, 2001).

Chapter Four: Week One: Grounded

1. Frank Hobbs and Nicole Stoops, "Demographic Trends in the 20th Century," *Census 2000 Special Reports,* November 2002, http://www.census.gov/prod/2002pubs/censr-4.pdf.

2. Anuradha Mittal, "Giving Away the Farm: The 2002 Farm Bill," Food First/Institute for Food and Development Policy, July 8, 2002, http://www.foodfirst.org/node/52.

3. The NPD Group, "Snacking in America 2008," http://www.npd.com/lps/PDF_SpecialReports/NPD_Snacking_America_TOC.pdf.

4. Steve Martinez, "Local Food Systems: Concepts, Impacts, and Issues," Economic Research Service of the U.S. Department of Agriculture, May 2010, http://www/ers.usda.gov/media/122864/en97_reportsummary_1_.pdf, accessed December 5, 2012.

Chapter Five: Week Two: Getting the Hang of It

1. Kelly M. Adams, Karen C. Lindell, Martin Kohlmeier, and Steven H. Zeisel, "Status of Nutrition Education in Medical Schools, *American Journal of Clinical*

Nutrition 83, no. 4 (April 2006): 941S–944S, http://www.ncbi.nlm.nih.gov/pmc/articles/PMC2430660/.

2. Barbara Bein, "Nutrition Education in U.S. Medical Schools 'Precarious,' Say Researchers," *American Academy of Family Physicians*, October 20, 2010, http://www.aafp.org/online/en/home/publications/news/news-now/resident-student -focus/20101020nutritioneduc.html.

3. Dictionary.com, *Columbia World of Quotations* (New York: Columbia University Press, 1996), http://quotes.dictionary.com/The_recommended_daily_requirement_for_ hugs_is_four. Here is another source: http://www.brainyquote.com/quotes/quotes/ v/virginiasa400866.html.

4. http://www.cdc.gov/foodsafety/rawmilk/raw-milk-questions-and-answers.html# related-outbreaks.

Chapter Six: Week Three: The Week of My Discontent

1. USDA Economic Research Service, last modified August 6, 2012, http://www .ers.usda.gov/data/fooddesert/about.html.

2. Charles Fishman, "A Farming Fairy Tale," *Fast Company,* May 2006, http:// www.fastcompany.com/56671/farming-fairy-tale.

3. "2012 World Hunger and Poverty Facts and Statistics," last modified December 4, 2011, http://www.worldhunger.org/articles/Learn/world%20hunger%20 facts%202002.htm#Does_the_world_produce_enough_food_to_feed_ everyone.

4. J. Putnam, J. Allshouse, and L. S. Kantor, "U.S. Per Capita Food Supply Trends," http://foodfarmsjobs.org/wp-content/uploads/2011/09/US-per-Capita-Food -Supply-Trends-More-Calories-Carbs-and-Fat.pdf.

5. Annette Clauson, "Despite Higher Food Prices, Percent of U.S. Income Spent on Food Remains Constant," *Amber Waves*, September 2008, http://www.ers .usda.gov/topics/food-nutrition-assistance/food-security-in-the-us.aspx.

Chapter Seven: Revelations of the Final Week

1. Anna Stern, "Saying Grace Around the World," February 13, 2009, *Yes!*, http:// www.yesmagazine.org/issues/food-for-everyone/saying-grace-around-the-world (illustrations by Nikki McClure not included).

Chapter Eight: Relational Eating

1. Thich Nhat Han, *Plum Village Chanting and Recitation Book* (Berkeley, CA: Parallax Press, June 2000).

2. Jonathan Bloom, *American Wasteland: How America Throws Away Nearly Half of Its Food (and What We Can Do About It)* (Cambridge, MA: Da Capo Lifelong Books, August 2011).

3. Michael E. Webber, "How to Make the Food System More Energy Efficient," *Scientific American*, December 29, 2011, http://www.scientificamerican.com/article.cfm?id=more-food-less-energy.

4. "Food Facts," Natural Resources Defense Council, September 2012, www.nrdc.org/living/eatingwell/files/foodwaste_2pgr.pdf.

5. Marian Nestle, quoted from an interview with Polly Hoppin of *The Project on Science and Public Policy*, accessed December 5, 2012, http://defendingscience.org/conversation-marion-nestle-phd.

6. Marine Conservation Society, *Good Fish Guide: The Consumer Guide to Sustainable Seafood*, accessed December 5, 2012, http://www.goodfishguide.co.uk.

7. Environmental Working Group, "2012 Shopper's Guide to Pesticides in Produce," accessed December 5, 2012, http://www.ewg.org/foodnews/summary/.

Chapter Nine: Bringing Our Eating Closer to Home

1. M. Fatih Citlak and Hüseyin Bingül, ed. *Rumi and His Sufi Path of Love* (Somerset, NJ: Tughra Books, 2007).

2. Community Food Security Coalition, *Whole Measures for Community Food Systems: Values-Based Planning and Evaluation*, 2009, http://foodsecurity.org/pub/WholeMeasuresCFS-web.pdf.

3. http://seattlefarmbillprinciples.org.

4. Steve Evans, King County Department of Natural Resources and Parks, "How much land is needed to feed King County's population?" *2009 Farms Report*, Appendix F, http://your.kingcounty.gov/dnrp/library/water-and-land/agriculture/future-of-farming/appendices/f-land-needed-to-feed-kc-population.pdf.

5. Michael Pollan, "Farmer in Chief," *New York Times*, October 9, 2008; http://www.nytimes.com/2008/10/12/magazine/12policy-t.html?pagewanted=all.

6. Niche Meat Processor Assistance Network, *State Poultry Processing Regulations*, August 2, 2012, http://www.extension.org/pages/33350/poultry-processing-regulations-and-exemptions.

7. http://localfoodshift.com/.

8. Growing Communities, accessed December 5, 2012, http://www.growingcommunities.org.

Index

activism:
  author's changing attitude toward, 225,
    250
  many lenses of, 317–18
  rebellion against industrial food system,
    243, 244
  by transformers, 294–96
agriculture:
  civic, 317
  industrial, 8, 52, 172, 175, 203, 236,
    244, 247
  preserving farmland, 247–48,
    268–69
  regional, 270
  relational, 301
  see also farmers
agro-ecological strategies, 280
Anderson, Anders and Bertine, 247
Anderson, Dorothy, 247–48
Anderson, Terra, 277–78
Anthes, Jacob, 92
anywhere eating, 17–18, 57–59, 223
apples, 116
Ashanti grace (Ghana), 219
Attwood, Maryon, 276–77, 315
autumn, reality of, 204–6

back-to-the-land movement, 28–32, 233
Bailey, Kimberly, 144, 145–46
beans, 72, 116
  baked bean recipe, 221
  cooking tips, 210
  hummus recipe, 26
Beckner, Tricia:
  cooking dinner for, 194–96
  and CSA garden, 44
  and 50 percent in 50 miles, 210, 261

food supplied by, 28, 56, 72, 75, 77, 88,
    97, 101, 105, 106, 117, 122, 148–49,
    156, 188, 189–90, 195, 224, 261
  and Kent, 44, 194–95, 313
  as market gardener, 44, 128–30, 213
  and relational eating, 223
  and 10-mile diet, 20–21, 47, 56, 66,
    88–89, 128
beets, 116
Belinda and Koren, 140–41, 198
  and chickens, 205, 261
  and milk, 71, 94, 130–33, 223
  and regulation, 131–32
belonging, 124, 226–27, 230
Berry, Wendell, 168, 312
big vs. small producers, see industrial food
    system
biodynamic farming, 244–45, 280
bioregions, 303–4
Bishop, Clark, 209
Bittman, Mark, 158, 160
blessings, 202, 218–20, 234–35, 312–13
Bloom, Jonathan, *American Wasteland*, 248
body, author's changing relationship with,
    224
Boin, Patrick, 52, 182, 184
Bradford, Jason, 251
Britt and Eric, *see* Conn, Britt and Eric
Brower, Claus, 67
Brown, Vicky, 313
  dessert cheese recipe, 86–87
  and Kickstarter, 251, 315
  and Little Brown Farm, 211, 315
  local cheese from, 101, 237–38
  and regulations, 238
Brownlee, Michael, 303
Brussels sprouts, recipe, 259

Buddhist grace, 218
butter, 114

caffeine, 74, 75
Callenbach, Ernest "Chick," 266–67
calories, 58, 178, 188, 189–90
Campbell, Colin, *Forks Over Knives,* 159
cancer:
    author's bout with, 12, 35, 199
    author's dream about, 263
    and diet, 64–65
    lessons learned from, 38–39
    and letting go, 39–40
canning food, 205–6
Carlin, George, 205
Carron, Laurie, 44
Center for a New American Dream, 39
Center for Whole Communities, 274
Chautauqua, 11–12
cheese, 57, 211
    goat (chèvre), 96–97
    recipes, 86–87, 221–22
    regulation of, 97, 237–38
Cherry, Lorna, 98–99
chicken, 160–61
    canning, 205–6, 261
    cost of, 156–58
    recipe, 184–86
children, 249–50
cholesterol, 188
Christian children's prayer, 219
"circle of we," 98
civic agriculture, 317
Coe, Helen, 93
coffee, 72, 213
comfort foods, 58
community:
    author's changing relationship
        with, 224
    belonging to, 226–27, 230
    food bank in, 77, 172–73
    food system for, 190, 274, 275, 303
    and Food 2020, 272–86
    freedom of, 312
    giving back to, 232
    and homecoming, 196–98, 224
    home cooking in, 97–98

    liberating, 201
    organizations within, 228–31
    and relational eating, 79, 227, 228–31,
        240, 246, 270, 298
    and Seattle Farm Bill, 287–88
    spirit of, 227, 228
    and 10-mile diet, 89, 105, 123, 124–30,
        198, 199
    Transition Towns, 49–50, 153–55
    trust in, 130
    volunteerism in, 228
community supported agriculture (CSA),
    44, 103, 189, 282
    becoming involved in, 166
    and relational eating, 4, 224, 240
compost, 129–30, 176, 232, 280
Concentrated Animal Feeding Operations
    (CAFOs), 169
Conlin, Richard, 286, 289, 290
Conn, Britt and Eric, 94–96, 168, 198
    family of, 314
    farmland of, 46, 94, 314
    income of, 213
    and local food system, 278, 313, 314
    permaculture method of, 94–95
    and relocalization, 41
    wedding of, 56, 66, 161, 223, 314
    and wheat crackers, 161
conscience, 169
conscious eating, 178–82
convection oven, 112, 118
convenience, 58
Conversation Cafés, 38, 39
conviviality, 192–94, 196
cooking from scratch, 115–16, 142–43
    author's relationship with, 121, 225
    beans and grains, 210
    benefits of, 139–42
    and food costs, 134–37
    mystical experience of, 124–30
    for others, 202
    recipes, *see* recipes
    signature soup, 143–44
    time involved in, 137–39
    tools of the trade, 118–20
Cooper, Ann, 249–50
co-ops, 237

cottage laws movement, 297
crunch, 111–13, 196
Cuba, 246
culture, 294

D'Adamo, Peter J., *Eat Right for Your Type*, 159
Dellinger, Drew, "Hieroglyphic Stairway," 37
Descartes, René, 197
diets and dieting, 14–16
  and cancer, 64–65
  and meat, 159, 180
  10 percent trick, 291
Dominguez, Joe, 37–38, 265
Dorcas and James, 101
Dowdell, Jess, 10, 252
  Basic Vegetable Stock, 107–9
  Bread and Butter Pickles, 27
  Coffee and Red Wine–Infused Lamb, 109–10
  Kale Chips, 145
  Local Bean Hummus, 26
  Nettle Soup, 85–86
  Parsnips and Aged Sheep Cheese Gratin, 221–22
  and Roaming Radish, 314–15
  seasonal menu by, 308–10
  sources of, 212, 213
  Squash Bisque, 260
Duwamish tribe, 68

Earth Day, 32–33
Ebey's Landing National Historical Reserve, 247
Ecocentric blog, 248
Ecological Footprint, 36
eggs, 210–11
80 percent fullness, 178
entitlement, author's changing attitude toward, 225
environment:
  exponential growth, 34–35
  limits to growth, 36–38
  overshoot and collapse, 35–36, 40
  and Peak Oil, 40–41, 153
Eric and Britt, *see* Conn, Britt and Eric

ethics, 58, 81–83, 171
ethylene gas, ripening with, 241
Exploring Island County's Food System, 277

fairness and justice, 274–75, 288
Fair Trade, 10, 167, 192, 213, 239, 257
Fallon, Sally, 146
family dinners, 193
Farm Bill, 165, 203, 287–88
farmers:
  average age of, 8, 281, 298
  co-ops, 237
  and Food 2020, 275
  making ends meet, 213
  relational, 236–39, 245, 248, 250, 301
  risks shouldered by, 215
  supporting, 168–69
  and sustainability, 164–67, 213, 215–16, 287
  tax breaks for, 280–81
  why they farm, 214–18
  young people as, 298–301
farmers' markets, 101–4
  and community, 126, 270
  and cottage laws movement, 297
  and 50-mile diet, 214
  and market gardeners, 43, 97, 103–4
  and relational eating, 236–37, 240, 252, 256
  researching, 83, 107
  sociability of, 6, 63, 101
  three-beeters at, 63, 303
farmland, preserving, 247–48, 268–69
FASS (fat, acid, salty, sweet), 122
fast food myths, 133–39
  costs of food, 134–37
  preparation time, 137–39
Feldman, Judy, 277
fertility, 244–45
50 percent within 50 miles, 155, 169, 204–6, 261, 271, 296
  canning food for, 205–6
  shopping list for, 206–14
fish, 73
Fisher, Rhiannon, 278
Fleming, Severine von Tscharner, 300–301

food:
    author's changing relationship with,
        224, 231
    canning, 205–6
    complexity of, 203
    costs of, 7, 72, 134–37, 156–58, 161,
        168, 179, 201, 238, 296
    donations of, 173
    emotionally charged, 203–4
    and fun, 204
    and the future, 47–49
    globally sourced, 239–40
    growing, 79–80, 144
    and love, 142, 202, 230–31, 232–33
    messages about, 25
    politics of, 203, 240, 244
    preferences vs. orthodoxies, 133
    small-scale vs. big producers, see
        industrial food system
    and sociability, 202
    at starting point, 78
    and waste, 248–49
Food, Conservation, and Energy Act
    (2008), 102
food-borne illnesses, 131, 238, 254
Food Charrette, 284–85
food democracy, 317
food deserts, 150
food drives, 173
food hubs, 251–52
food journal, 180
Food Lifeline, 172
food map, 272–74, 293–94, 302–4
food miles, 17, 95, 123, 241, 270–72, 304
food sheds, 122, 153, 213, 285, 303–4,
    307–8
food stories, 23–25
food system:
    agenda for eaters in, 296
    being our own, 4, 202–3, 231
    benefits of, 169–72
    community, 190, 274, 275, 303
    complementary, 290–91
    elements of, 293–94
    and February 50/50, 207
    health-centered, 287
    household, 302

    industrial, see industrial food system
    mapping, 272–74, 293–94, 302–4
    and natural world, 125, 306–7, 317
    participatory, 317
    person-to-person, 238–39
    rebellion against, 243, 244
    regional, 303–4
    relational, see relational eating
    transformers in, 294–96
food technologies, 203
Food 2020, 272–86
    back casting in, 281, 284
    communities in, 275
    effects of, 282
    goal of, 278
    healthy people in, 275
    how to do it, 282–85
    invitation to, 283–84
    justice and fairness in, 274–75
    and local economy, 276
    mapping your system, 272–74
    meeting for planning of, 278–81
    progress in, 288–90
    sustainable ecosystems in, 275
    vibrant farms in, 275
food value chain, 294
freedom, 244, 312
free range, 160
Fresh Food for the Table, 282
freshness, 241
frugality, 57–58, 59, 63, 243

Gerber, Georgia, 258
Gibbons, Euell, 30
GI Bill, 299
Gleeful Gleaners, 77, 229
Globescope Pacific Assembly (1989), 33–34
goat leg, 141–42, 223
Good Cheer Food Bank, 77, 172–73,
    228–29, 282, 316
Goose Community Grocery Store, 61–62
government controls, 168, 237–39, 304
    on cheese, 97, 237–38
    on eggs, 210–11
    on milk, 70, 131–32, 203, 316–17
    scale-appropriate, 297–98, 317
government subsidies, 169, 238

grace, 202, 218–20, 234–35
grains, 161–63, 209–10
gratitude, 232, 234–36
Gray, Farmer, 30
Gray, Pat, 30
Greenbank Farm Training Center, 229, 277, 279, 281, 315–16
Greenhorns, 300–301
Green Revolution, 203
Growing Communities (UK), 304–6
growth:
    exponential, 34–35
    limits to, 36–38

Halprin, Anna, 311–12
hara hachi bu (80 percent full), 178
Hayes, Denis, 32
health, 58, 139–40, 275
Helsing Farm, Chehalis, 103
herbs and spices, 74, 75, 117–18
Hindu grace (India), 219
Hippocrates, 118
homecoming, 196–98, 224
homegrown food, 144
honey, 71
hope, 4–5, 264–67, 269, 270, 276, 277, 282, 292
Hopkins, Rob, 42, 49
horizontal distribution, 269–71
household food system, 302
Hubbard, Lauren, 208, 209, 261
hunger, 15, 203
hunter-gatherer lifestyle, 41

Imes, Loren and Patty, 212–13
industrial food system:
    and agriculture, 8, 52, 172, 175, 203, 236, 244, 247
    dependence on, 3, 171–72, 201, 244, 269
    efficacy of, 124, 134, 169–72, 178, 190
    and ethics, 58, 171
    and food-borne disease, 238, 254
    hidden costs of, 201, 242–43, 248, 257
    impersonal, 4, 89, 225, 240
    leaving it to the experts, 201
    and obesity, 232

and oil, 40, 52, 245
and price, 7, 72, 157–58, 161, 168, 179, 238, 296
and regulations, 8, 72, 168, 211, 237–39, 251, 296, 297–98, 317
relational eating vs., 224, 230, 232, 237, 240
trend toward, 99, 135, 139, 179
vs. the little guy, 8, 72, 97, 157–58, 172, 174, 175, 237, 250, 269, 295
integrity, 232

Jesperson, Annie, 217–18, 316
Jewish grace, 220
journal, keeping, 180
Jurriaans, Sieb, 258, 259
justice and fairness, 274–75, 288

Kahn, Gene, 173–77, 268
kale, 115–16
Kale Chips, recipe, 145
Katz, Rebecca, *One Bite at a Time,* 121–22
Kerr, Graham, 119–20
Kickstarter, 251, 315
King, F. H., 176
Klinenberg, Eric, *Going Solo,* 193
Kohlmeier, Martin, 117
Korrow, Chris, 248, 264, 316
Krapfel, Paul, *Shifting,* 285–86

lamb, recipe, 109–10
Langley, Washington, 93
Langley Middle School garden, 229
Lao-Tzu, 36
Lappé, Frances Moore and Anna, ix–xii, 168
Lazarus, Karen, 277, 278
LeBaron, Duke and Kate, 233–34
lemons and limes, 74
letting go, 39–40
liberating limits, 198–201
Lobell, Robbie, 315
local:
    expanding to everyone, 268, 270
    and horizontal distribution, 269–71
    relationships in, 153–55
    shopping criteria, 257–58

local (*cont.*)
 USDA definition of, 102, 270
 vs. big food producers, *see* industrial food system
 wherever you are, 153–55, 239–40
 your version of, 307–8
local eating:
 effects of, 6–10
 and farmland preservation, 247–48, 268–69
 and fertility, 244–45
 and freshness, 241
 and frugality, 243
 and the future, 250–53
 hyperlocal (10 miles), 47
 is it for you?, 5–6
 and local prosperity, 246
 rare practice of, 163–67
 reasons to do it, 6, 240–53, 254–55
 rebellion, 243, 244
 relational, 153, 240–53
 and relocalization, 9–10
 in restaurants, 212
 and ripeness, 241
 and security, 245–46
 and subsidiarity, 191–92
 and taste, 242
 where to begin, 256–57
 and wholesomeness, 242–43
Local Investing Opportunity Network (LION), 251, 314
location, 106–7
Long, Joe, 67
Long, Nancy, 67
Long Family Farm, 66–67, 69, 223, 224
love:
 and biodynamic farming, 244
 cooking with, 142, 206, 308
 food is love, 142, 202, 230–31, 232–33
 and local food, 8, 89, 101, 122, 223, 232–33, 240, 253
 need for, 231
 pride vs., 153
 and 10-mile diet, 15, 16, 105, 142, 191, 199, 202

 and vulnerability, 127
 and web of life, 226
Lower Skagit First Nations people, 11

Mackies (settlers), 12
Marin Agricultural Land Trust, California, 247
Marshall Plan, 299
Marty and Beulah, 30–31
Meadows, Donella, 58
meat:
 Bittman's views on, 158–61
 at custom-cut slaughterhouses, 297
 living with less, 291–92
 from Long Family Farm, 66–67, 69, 223, 224
 meatloaf recipe, 51
 no-meat mantra, 182
 raising your own, 291–92
 scale-appropriate regulations for, 297–98, 317
 and 10 percent rule, 181
 as treat, 180–81
 trends away from, 180–82
meatless Mondays, 181
Menominee Indians, 31
menu, seasonal, 308–10
migrant farmworkers, 163
milk:
 author's quest for, 69–71, 89, 90–91, 94, 97, 223
 goat, 69–71, 97
 pasteurized, 70
 raw, 70, 130–33, 203, 297
 regulation of, 70, 131–32, 203, 316–17
Miller, Rhea, 284–85
Mitchell, Pam, 198
 and farmers' markets, 101–4
 food calculation by, 43, 45, 172
 as market gardener, 103–4, 216, 314
 and SPIN-Gardening, 43–45
Mobley, Neal, 101
moderation, 153
Molly's Season Extender CSA, 72
monocropping, 190, 242
Monroe, Marilyn, 16
moral issues, 171

Morrill, Lisa, 50–52
Morris, Kimmer, 249
multistakeholder dialogue, 276
Muzzall, Ron and Shelly, 212

Nattress, Vincent, 50, 52
natural food, 105–6, 122–24
natural world, 90, 125, 167, 306–7, 317
Nelson, Gaylord, 32
Nelson, Willie, 197
Nestle, Marian, 249
New Road Map Foundation, 59
Nichols, Mike (food delivery), 207–8, 270
Niemuller, Martin, 307
night soil, 176
Nina (cheese lady), 97, 141, 198, 211
Now It's Your Turn:
    conscious eating, 178–82
    cooking, 142–43
    dining together, 218
    establish your home base, 78
    food ethic, 81–83
    food journal, 180
    food messages, 25
    graces, 218–20
    grow your own, 79–80
    host a Potluck with a Purpose, 83–85
    how to start a Transition Town group, 49–50
    location, 106–7
    motivation, 78–79, 254–55
    shopping criteria, 257–58
    tasks, 308
    tell your food stories, 23–25
    treasure hunt, 83
    where to begin, 256–57
    your food future, 47–49
    your life as an eater, 22–23
    your version of "local," 307–8
    your "where", 79
nuts, 89–90

obesity, 232
oil (cooking), 74

oil (petroleum):
    and industrial food system, 40, 52, 245
    peak, 40–41, 52, 68, 93, 153, 255
    price of, 280
omega-3 oils, 74
organic food, 167, 280
    laws governing, 211
    scaling up, 268
Organic Valley Dairy Cooperative, 16
overeating, 19
overshoot and collapse, 35–36, 40

Pachamama Awakening the Dreamer Symposium, 38
Peak Oil, 40–41, 52, 68, 93, 153, 255
Penguin Companion to Food, 124, 125
permaculture, 94–95, 280
Peterson, Cary, 229, 243, 316
Peterson, Molly and John, 72, 198, 217, 224, 261, 313, 316
pickles, recipes, 27
pink slime, 250
plate size, 178–79
potatoes, 116
potlatch, 98–99
Potlucks with a Purpose, 65–66, 77, 83–85
preference, 58
pressure cooker, 120, 143
Putnam, Robert, *Bowling Alone,* 98

querencia (longing for home), 187
Quinn, Daniel, 99

Ranker, Kevin, 316
Ratekin, Kent, 44, 89, 105, 194–95, 213, 313
rebellion, 243, 244
recipes:
    Basic Vegetable Stock, 107–9
    Bread and Butter Pickles, 27
    Chanterelle and Cauliflower Mushroom–Stuffed Roasted Chicken Breast, 184–86
    Chef Sibrand Jurriaans Brussels Sprouts, 259
    Georgie's Grandma Smith's Rockwell Baked Beans, 221

recipes (*cont.*)
  Grass-Fed Bone Marrow Broth,
    146–47
  Jess Dowdell's Nettle Soup, 85–86
  Jess's Coffee and Red Wine–Infused
    Lamb, 109–10
  Jess's Parsnip and Aged Sheep Cheese
    Gratin, 221–22
  Kale Chips, 145
  Local Bean Hummus, 26
  Ma's Meatloaf, 51
  Nutty Renee's Red Kuri Soup, 183–84
  Root Chips, 145
  Salad of Fall Greens, Poached Hen's
    Egg, Walnut Vinaigrette, 53–55
  Squash Bisque by Jess Dowdell, 260
  Sweet Pickle Relish, 27
  Vicky Brown's Dessert Cheese, 86–87
  your signature soup, 143–44
relational eating, 124–30, 223–40
  author's movement into, 26, 89, 192,
    201, 223, 224–25, 250, 261
  and belonging, 226–27, 230
  and children, 249–50
  and community, 79, 227, 228–31, 240,
    246, 270, 298
  and cooking, 124, 142, 225, 308
  definitions of, 4, 9, 192, 226, 253, 271
  eating together, 234–36
  and exotics, 239–40
  and farmers' markets, 236–37, 240,
    252, 256
  and farming, 236–39, 245, 248, 250,
    301
  food and love, 230–31, 232–33
  and food value chain, 294
  and the future, 250–53, 267–69
  and global food sources, 239–40
  and gratitude, 232, 234–36
  and hope, 269, 270, 276, 277
  and horizontal distribution, 269–71
  and integrity, 232
  and local eating, *see* local eating
  and sprouting, 79–80
  vs. industrial food system, 224, 230,
    232, 237, 240
  web of eating, 127, 225–26
    web of life, 226, 232, 234, 239–40, 253,
      307
relocalization:
  author's commitment to, 46, 226, 264
  and local finance, 314
  movement, 5, 9–10, 40–41, 50, 85
  and Transition Town, 42–43, 154–55,
    303
resilience, 9, 154, 289, 290, 293
resourcefulness, 140, 154
Rhinelander commune, 28–32, 206
Ridenour, Laura, 317
ripeness, 241
Robbins, John, *Diet for a New America,* 58,
  159, 168
Root Chips recipe, 145
Roth, Geneen, 230–31
  Women Food and God, 231

salad recipe, 53–55
Salish people, 11
salt, 74
Sandra, 198
  goat leg from, 141–42, 223
Satir, Virginia, 123
sauerkraut, 134
scalability, 176–77
scale-appropriate regulations, 297–98, 317
scaling up, 268–69
school lunches, 249–50
Schuman, Michael, 303
seasonal harvests, 165
Seattle:
  Farm Bill principles, 287–88
  food evolution in, 286–90
security, 245–46
self-sufficiency, 46, 192–94
September Eat Local Challenge, 77
serotiny, 292–93
Shaw, George Bernard, 36
shopping, 59–63, 257–58
Shulman, Phyllis, 286, 288–89, 290
Silby, Georgina, 208–9, 216–17, 224, 238,
  261
simplicity, 57
Singer, Jean, 277, 278
Sioux grace, 220

slowing down, 179
Smith, Georgie, 198, 314
    baked bean recipe, 220–21
    heirloom beans from, 72, 224, 238, 261
    as market gardener, 207, 208
    reasons to farm, 215–16
    and Willowwood Farm, 182–83
Snacking in America (NPD), 100
Snohomish tribe, 68
Snoqualmie tribe, 68
solo lifestyle, 192–94
soups:
    Basic Vegetable Stock, 107–9
    Bone Marrow Broth, 146–47
    Nettle Soup, 85–86
    Red Kuri Soup, 183–84
    Squash Bisque, 260
    your signature recipe, 143–44
South Whidbey, 92–93, 98–100
Spangle, Linda, 113
spices and herbs, 74, 75, 117–18
SPIN-Gardening, 43–45
Squash Bisque, recipe, 260
Star Store, Langley, 59–61, 71–72
Steele, Carolyn, *Hungry City*, 68
Steiner, Rudolf, 44, 195
Stoll, Andrew, 74
subsidiarity, 191–92
sustainability, 168, 177, 250
    conference (1989) on, 33–34
    and exponential growth, 34–35
    as extreme sport, 21–22, 95, 155, 223,
        243, 291, 312
    and farmers, 164–67, 213, 215–16, 287
    and Food 2020, 275
    and limits to growth, 36–38
    and overshoot and collapse, 35–36, 40
    and survival, 41–43
sustainable development, 286
Sustainable Seattle, 39
Sustainable Whidbey Coalition, 95
Swanson, Lynn, 237
sweeties, 113

Talbot, Nathaniel, 316
taste buds, 125, 179, 242
Tata corporation, 77

TED talks, 158–60, 191
10-mile diet, 1–2
    author's blogs about, 75–76, 92, 106,
        128–30, 142, 172, 191–92, 262
    author's lifestyle changes in, 190–91
    beginning of, 20–21, 28, 56–57
    constraints of, 149–50, 198–201
    continuing with, 223
    D-Day minus 1, 88–89
    effects of, 3, 105, 123, 188–91, 199,
        224–25, 311–12
    end of, 196
    expanding the definition of, 155
    food miles, 123
    food rules derived from, 202–4
    mystical experience of, 124–30
    practicalities of, 128
    solitary eating in, 192–94, 196
    and Transition Town gathering, 149–55
    Week One: Grounded!, 88–110
    Week Two: Getting the Hang of It,
        111–47
    Week Three: The Week of My
        Discontent, 148–86
    Week Four: Final Week, 187–222
    wherever you are, 153–55
Teresa, Mother, grace of, 219
Thistlewaite, Rebecca, "So You Say You
        Want a Food Revolution," 163–67,
        168
Thoreau, Henry, 32
time, value of, 200–201
time limitations, 137–39, 193
Tobey (chickens), 156–58, 168, 194, 224
togetherness, 140, 218, 234–36
Trader Joe's, 61–62
transformations, 224–25
transformers, 294–96
Transition Colorado, 303
Transition Town:
    gathering, 149–55
    how to start, 49–50
    and relocalization, 42–43, 154–55, 303
Transition Whatcom County, 152
Transition Whidbey, 65–66, 77, 83, 93,
        229, 272
Tree Top Bakers, 101

trust, 130, 293
turnips, 75–76
Twain, Mark, 153

Vallat, Gary, 233
Van's Produce, Seattle, 62, 77
victory gardens, 291
volunteerism, 228

Waldorf education, 44
waste, 248–49
Waters, Alice, 212, 249
web of eating, 127, 225–26
web of life:
    awareness of, 203
    being woven into, 318
    and relational eating, 226, 232, 234,
        239–40, 253, 307
weight loss, 188
wheat, 161–63
Whidbey Institute, 229
Whidbey Island:
    ability to feed itself, 45, 46, 67, 189,
        279–80
    community of, 45
    Food 2020 in, 272–86
    map, iv
    native tribes of, 68
Whidbey Island Farm Tour menu, 308–10
"Whidbey Island Grown" brand, 239, 276

Whidbey Island Local Compost (WILC),
    280, 281
Whidbey Island Local Lending (W.I.L.L.),
    251, 282
Whidbey Island Nourishes (W.I.N.),
    229–30
Whidbey Island Slow Food Convivium, 52
Whidbey Island Winery, 71–72
Whitney, John and Else, 210–11
whole foods, 182, 242
whole-foods Lent, 180, 242
Whole Measures for Community Food
    Systems, 274–76
wholesomeness, 242–43
Wicks, Judy, 212
Wildenson, Percy, 67
Willeford, Lynn, 314
Wolfe, Chris, 152–54, 223
women, economic independence of,
    193

Yes! magazine, 191
Young, John, 198
young farmers, encouraging, 298–301
Your Money or Your Life (Robin and
    Dominguez), 37–38, 46, 57, 138

zackers, 111–12
zookies, 114
zucchini, 111, 115, 118